YOGA FOR EVERY BODY

A beginner's guide to the practice of postures, breathing exercises and meditation

LUISA RAY

Illustrations by

Angus Sutherland

To everybody who is yet to take the first step.

A QUICK THANK YOU

It's so hard to fit everything you want to into one book! As as special thank you to my readers, I've put together 2 extra books to help you along your yoga journey.

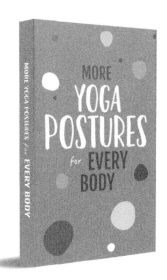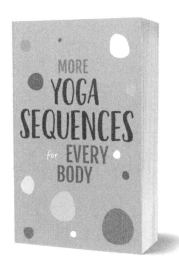

Get FREE unlimited access to these books, and all my future releases by joining our community.

SCAN WITH YOUR CAMERA TO JOIN!

CONTENTS

INTRODUCTION

Many years ago, when I had just finished university, I hit a turning point. I didn't know what to do with myself. I had been in school and studying for almost my whole life, and I had a hard time adjusting to moving on in the outside world. It wasn't just an uncertainty about what career path to start down, it was something more fundamental. All my friends and contemporaries seemed to know exactly what they wanted to do and where they wanted to go - and they were doing it. But somehow, I didn't, and I wasn't. I felt stuck.

It got worse. I became anxious, and overstressed. I started to suffer from depression. It became debilitating. For weeks I didn't want to leave the house, or even to get out of bed. I missed job interviews that I applied for, then I stopped applying for them at all. I saw opportunities slipping away from me, but I couldn't make myself do anything about it. Nothing seemed worthwhile. I couldn't see my place in the world and was beginning to feel that I shouldn't be in it.

This isn't an uncommon situation. I know now that I wasn't unusual, but at the time I didn't realise it. Back then, people were less willing and more rarely talked to others about their mental health. It's getting a bit better now, but it's still a difficult topic. I'm lucky - lucky enough to have had a college education, lucky enough to have a supportive family who could afford for me to continue to live at home. This isn't the case for everyone. At the time, I also realised this and it only made my mental state worse.

It was a girlfriend who convinced me to go to a yoga class with her. She had to drag me there. The effect was immediate, but the results took a long time. I felt as though in a dark sea of pain and confusion, someone had thrown me a lifeline. I wasn't on dry land yet, I still had to hold on and find my way out, but now I knew for sure that there was a way out.

Since then, I haven't looked back.

I've stuck with yoga longer than anything else in my life, and my whole life has changed.

I'm not telling you this story so that you'll feel sorry for me. Above all: this book isn't about me; this book is about you.

That's just the route that took me to yoga. Yours might be similar. Most likely it will be different. Life offers up all sorts of challenges: pits for us to fall down and valleys for us to cross. Everyone will have health problems at some point – whether they're physical or mental – it's part of the price of being human. You'll find yourself facing all sorts of turning points in your life. If you've found this book, I hope it can convince you to make a start on the life-altering path of yoga and provide you with a guide to taking some of the steps.

It was after several careers and after attending several yoga teacher trainings that I decided to write this book. I've been teaching yoga for many years, and the people who come to the classes in the big city yoga studios look predominantly the same. It's self-selecting, the people who look like the pictures of people doing yoga postures in magazines and on the internet, are the ones who come into the studios. The studios are located in affluent areas, and the people coming to class are from the surrounding neighbourhoods.

It's the people who are in good shape and who can afford the membership fees who are going to class.

Almost everyone's heard of yoga, and although more

and more people are practising it, some of the people it would benefit the most - who need it the most - are not doing it.

And although it's been around for a long time, in the last few decades it's become incredibly popular. There are more and more yoga studios opening, new apps and platforms being developed daily and countless pictures of people balancing serenely in advanced postures against the sunsets of social media.

It can be a bit overwhelming. There are so many different styles and so many different opinions it can be hard to know where to start.

The aim of this book is to take away some of that confusion.

Ultimately it only matters that you practise the kind of yoga that's right for you, and you are the only person who can tell what that is.

Yoga is a path to understanding yourself better, and living in your world more fully, and by reading this you're making a very important step on that journey. It's a journey that can last you a lifetime, a journey that can change your life, like it changed mine, and lead you to amazing and unexpected places.

PART 1

YOGA IS FOR YOU

CHAPTER 1
WHAT CAN YOGA DO?

Before even trying it for the first time, often the first question someone will ask is: "Why should I do yoga?" If you've never done it before you might be thinking the same thing. If you've already started, maybe you asked the same question once upon a time. You've only got so many hours in your day, and you've got a lot of things to do. Why do this in particular? What can it actually do? And will it even work the way its meant to?

Everyone has a different idea of what it means to "do yoga." Some people even say that yoga isn't something you can "do," instead they say that it is a state of consciousness that you can reach. It is a state of connection between you and fundamental forces that generate and run the universe that we all inhabit.

Compared to how you feel on a day-to-day basis, the ups and downs inherent to life, that state might seem like it's a long way off. If it sounds like too big a step to start with, don't worry. We're going to start small.

The yoga that you're going to learn in this book is a set of physical postures, breathing exercises and relaxation techniques. Practising these movements and techniques can have a profound effect on your physical wellbeing and mental health.

You can improve your flexibility, reduce stress, strengthen your body, sleep better, feel great, live a vibrant life and much more.

WHERE DOES IT ALL COME FROM?

This kind of modern yoga developed out of a South Asian cultural and spiritual tradition with deep roots and many branches. Some claim that it could be up to five thousand years old. It's hard to track down where it comes from beyond the written record. Over the generations of its practice, it has been reinterpreted and reimagined as different ideas and methods have been incorporated into it.

It's beyond the scope of this book to go into the depths of this tradition, and there are many great resources which can help you understand the history and development of yoga. By practising it you may be inspired to seek further knowledge.

Sometimes this kind of yoga is referred to as Hatha Yoga, often when it is being counterposed against the most popular "brands" of yoga: Ashtanga, Bikram, Iyengar, Power or Yin, to name just a few. The truth is that all modern postural yoga, all the big well-known systems, are themselves an offshoot of the branch of Hatha Yoga.

So, whether you do fast yoga or slow yoga, gentle yoga or hard yoga, beginners' yoga or advanced yoga, it is all a kind of Hatha Yoga.

In the simplest of terms, Hatha Yoga focuses on the transformation of physical and mental energy.

WHAT DOES THE SCIENCE SAY?

When yoga entered the mainstream in the West, tales of its life-changing effects came with it, and since then research has tried to keep up.

Studies have been done to assess the effects of practising yoga and the results are amazing. If you want to explore more of the research, have a look at the references at the back of the book. Here's a long list of all the scientifically proven things that you can do.

Yoga can:

REDUCE STRESS:
Many studies have shown that practising yoga can reduce the production of cortisol, the primary stress hormone in the body.

RELIEVE ANXIETY:
Multiple studies have shown that yoga practice can reduce feelings of anxiety. Not only has yoga been shown to be better at reducing anxiety than other physical activities like walking, but it has also been shown to reduce the severe anxiety that conditions like post-traumatic stress disorder can generate.

REDUCE INFLAMMATION:
Inflammation is a normal immune response, but when it gets out of control, it is at the centre of so many physical and mental ailments: heart disease, diabetes and cancer are all pro-inflammatory diseases. Yoga may be able to protect against certain diseases caused by chronic inflammation.

FIGHT DEPRESSION:
Studies have shown that yoga can be a great complementary therapy to the traditional treatments for depression. Reducing cortisol levels influences levels of serotonin in the brain, the neurotransmitter often associated with depression. Some research has shown that it can even be effective for people with depression that has not responded well to antidepressants.

PREVENT HEART DISEASE:
Studies have shown that yoga can improve the health of your heart. Practising yoga can lower your blood pressure, an important risk factor for heart disease. Other studies have also shown that yoga can slow the progression of heart disease from those already suffering from it.

DECREASE LOWER BACK PAIN:
Lower back pain affects so many people at some point during their life and it can be debilitating. It can prevent you from working, exercising and sleeping. Practising yoga can provide lower back pain relief and an improvement in back-related function - some research

even suggests that yoga is just as effective at relieving back pain as physical therapy.

REDUCE CHRONIC PAIN:
It turns out that yoga can help many types of chronic pain, not just lower back pain. Practised therapeutically, research has shown it to have decreased the pain and improved the physical function of different individuals suffering from carpal tunnel syndrome and osteoarthritis of the knee.

IMPROVE SLEEP QUALITY:
Studies show that incorporating yoga into your routine could help promote better sleep. One possible way this happens is due to melatonin, a hormone that regulates sleep and wakefulness - yoga has been shown to increase the secretion of this important hormone.

IMPROVE FLEXIBILITY AND BALANCE:
This is the obvious one - this is often why people include yoga in their routine in the first place. The science backs it up - even practising 15 minutes a day could make a big difference if you're looking to enhance performance by increasing flexibility and balance.

INCREASE STRENGTH:
This is also an obvious one once you try some of the postures, in particular the sun salutations and arm balances. Research has demonstrated a significant increase in upper body strength, endurance and weight loss (although the participants of one study did do 24 sun salutes a day, 6 days a week for 24 weeks, which is quite a lot of sun salutations - especially if you're just starting out!)

HELP IMPROVE BREATHING:
This can be especially important for those with lung disease, heart problems and asthma. Research has shown that a combination of yoga and breathing exercises can improve the lungs vital capacity, which is a measure of the maximum amount of air that can be expelled from the lungs.

IMPROVE DIGESTION:
When your body is continually stuck in a stress response, the nervous system interferes with the body's

ability to digest food. The sympathetic nervous system diverts energy away from processes like digestion. Research has linked relaxation therapies, like the kind of progressive muscle relaxation you might do at the end of a practice, with improvements to gastrointestinal function.

HELP WITH WEIGHT MANAGEMENT:
If this is something you're working on, the exercise aspect of yoga can clearly help with weight loss, but surprisingly, so can the relaxation part. Some studies have linked a high secretion of the stress hormone, cortisol, with an increase in abdominal fat. Reducing stress can help to target this.

WHAT YOGA ISN'T

This might seem like a strange subject but it's an important one. So many people have an idea in their mind about what yoga might be before even trying it. At best this leads to confusion. At worst it can put you off stepping onto a yoga mat in the first place.

So here is a list of yoga myths that need debunking.

MYTH #1: YOGA IS ONLY FOR THE FLEXIBLE.
This just doesn't make any sense. As you'll have just read in the previous section, yoga can help improve flexibility - so much research has proven it. In fact, although some parts of yoga might be easier if you're flexible, some parts might be a lot harder. The cliché that's always used by yoga teachers is: "Saying you're not flexible enough to practise yoga is like saying you're too dirty to take a bath."

MYTH #2: YOGA IS A RELIGION.
Yoga grew up around a religion - or maybe it was vice versa - the religion grew up around yoga, but yoga itself is not a religion. If you have religious beliefs of any sort, if anything it might help you to understand them better. If you don't, it might make you think about yourself and your position in the universe, which is fundamentally at the heart of the philosophy, and might help you to understand that better too.

MYTH #3: YOU MUST BE VEGETARIAN OR VEGAN TO PRACTISE YOGA.

You can eat anything you want and drink anything you like, and you'll still get a huge amount of benefit from practising yoga postures, doing breathing exercises and meditating. If you dive deeper into the philosophy of yoga you might start to question your choices and think about how your actions affect others, and this might lead you to vegetarianism. No one will try to make you become vegetarian or vegan, and anyone who does is pushing their own agenda.

MYTH #4: YOGA IS ONLY ABOUT STRETCHING.

If that's your impression of yoga, then think again. Try practising Crow pose, or holding Low-level plank, and you'll see straight away that yoga can be about strength as well as stretching! Long-term healthy movement requires a balance of strength and flexibility, which over time yoga will build.

MYTH #5: YOGA IS TOO EASY.

If you're a dedicated workout fanatic who loves HIIT and extreme sports, you might be under the impression that yoga looks very easy. You move slowly, you don't have to lift heavy weights. While some aspects of it will be easy compared to doing pull ups and deadlifts, for instance, some parts will be challenging. In fact, no matter what your background is, you're very likely to find something you can't do straight away in a yoga practice - whether it's a physical posture, or just staying still for a few moments.

MYTH #6: YOGA IS TOO HARD.

If you've been out of action for a long time, or your muscles feel really tight, or you don't move much or you hate stretching, you might feel that yoga is just too hard. The great thing about learning yoga yourself is that you can start simply. Yoga is as hard as you make it. If you want to practise slow gentle stretches, that's fine. If you just want to work on breathing exercises, that's fine too. Once you get started, you'll find that both your capacity and your perception of what's difficult and what's easy will change.

MYTH #7: YOGA IS NOT FOR MEN.

This is often combined with myth #1 - usually from the mouths of men who don't want to try yoga. In the past, yoga postures in the format that we've come to practise now were almost exclusively practised by men. So historically, yoga definitely was for men. Nowadays, although yoga is often marketed at women through clothing and lifestyle brands, the number of male professional athletes who practise yoga keeps on increasing. Stars from almost every sport have taken up the practice and it has prolonged their careers.

CHAPTER 2
YOGA IS FOR EVERY BODY

This is a short chapter, but it's a very important one, perhaps the most important chapter in the book.

You don't need to look a certain way to practise yoga. Regardless of the images that are displayed all over the internet, you don't need to be a certain shape, size, gender, race or age to do yoga. You don't need to be bendier than a pretzel or strong enough to balance on your hands. You don't have to look like you've just stepped out of a spa, or that you're so calm and zen that nothing could shake you, you don't have to be young and fit, or have chakra tattoos, or prayer necklaces, or carry a yoga mat with you wherever you go. Anybody can do yoga, and it is for every type of body.

In fact, the postures don't even need to look a certain way. The pictures in this book are just a reference, a guide that will help you find your own true alignment.

YOUR UNIQUE ANATOMY

You are unique. Everything about you is different from anybody else on the entire planet. On the outside that's obvious: your features, your body parts, your skin colour and your hairstyle are all unique to you

Internally you're unique as well. Although humans are all built on roughly the same pattern, we're not the same.

Inside everything's different. That means the number and shape of your bones, and how they fit together, the structure and integration of your muscles, the places where your body naturally accumulates fat and the type of connective tissue that joins everything together. It's all different. There's more of course, but on a physical level, the degree of variation between people is immense.

And you've had a different life from everyone else too. You learnt to walk and to run and move in your own time, you played different games when you were little, different sports and activities when you were at school, you've done different kinds of work throughout your life. How your brain and your body work together is incalculably complex and is the thing that makes you YOU.

This all means that your yoga practice will be unique to you.

YOUR UNIQUE LIFESTYLE

Yoga can change your life, but your life needs to have space for yoga.

Everybody's life is different: you might have a busy work schedule, childcare responsibilities, endless commitments and a packed social life. You might be between jobs and have some spare hours in the middle of the day. You might be going through a change of pace and need help speeding up or slowing down.

Your life is unique, and you should live it how you want to.

The good thing is there's no fixed model that your yoga practice must resemble. You can fit yoga into your life no matter what shape it takes. If that means it's just five minutes in the morning or a whole hour in the evening, it doesn't matter. The important thing is to do what you can.

CHAPTER 3
HOW TO USE THIS BOOK

VIDEO KILLED THE RADIO STAR

...and pretty much every other kind of star out there...

There are so many YouTube tutorials, Instagram clips and yoga platforms that offer videos to help you with your yoga practice. There are so many out there that it's easy to think they're the best way of learning how to practise yoga. That's exactly why you need this book. While videos can be a very valuable teaching and learning tool, they're not ideal.

There are two big problems.

The first problem doesn't really have anything to do with the videos themselves, but rather the context they're in. You'll probably watch whatever you're watching or streaming on your phone, which means it's very easy to get distracted by all the other amazing things that are also on your phone (like the social media app that the video was on in the first place, or the message that pinged up just as you were about to go into Dead body pose...).

What might have been a productive yoga practice turns into 25 minutes of scrolling or a reel of automatically recommended videos once the 3-minute tutorial ends. That might leave you more distracted than you would have been if you hadn't tried practising yoga in the first place.

The second problem is that videos can be too absorbing. This might seem like a good thing - the more absorbing, the more exposure you have to the information. And while it might mean that you grasp some of the information more quickly, it will also mean that you are not in the best mental state to practise yoga. There's too much sensory input. You can easily be overloaded.

Of course it will be more time consuming to read the book, practise a few postures, then go back to the book to see if you'll get a better understanding of what you're trying to do. However, it will mean that while you're actually doing the postures, you're not looking at images of someone else. In other words, your attention won't be diverted to the external world, and you can start to focus on internal experience.

And this is a really important point: we spend so much of our lives comparing ourselves to others or basing our sense of value on how we look, that it's crucial that we can find space in your day away from those impulses. Yoga is something that can create that space.

If you're brand new to yoga, one of the best things you can do is to sit on your mat with this book and slowly work your way through some of the postures.

GET YOURSELF TO CLASS

This book isn't designed to replace a real-life yoga teacher. However, if there aren't any yoga teachers where you live, then a book like this will be the best alternative.

The best yoga teachers will help you to understand that ultimately you are your own best teacher. They will try to help you realise that yoga is a process of self-exploration and self-inquiry that can be done in many different ways. If they insist that you practise exactly a certain way and claim that their way is the only way to have success in yoga, it's quite likely that they're trying to create a relationship where you're dependent on their teaching to feel fulfilled in your practice. This is the kind of student-teacher relationship that you want to avoid.

Practising with a yoga teacher in a public class or on a one-to-one basis is a totally different experience from practising on your own and is one that can have so many physical and mental benefits. It's well worth doing.

However, yoga practice works best when you can do it regularly - daily if possible - and getting to a class in a yoga studio every day is a huge commitment of time and money. It's not always possible. So, it's also well worth learning how to do it for yourself as well.

Use this book to establish a practice that you can do at home, anytime, regardless of what else you've got in your day. If that means it's 15 minutes in the morning before you've had a shower, or last thing at night before you go to bed, that's fine.

It doesn't mean you shouldn't try to go to a yoga class. Yoga is a lifelong learning experience, and the more resources you have, the better. Always leave yourself open to new learning.

WRITING YOUR OWN INSTRUCTIONS MANUAL

On one level, yoga practice can help you do that. It can help you understand how you operate physically and mentally. Of course, you don't have to do it literally. You don't have to write anything out.

Before you practise a posture or a sequence, make sure you read through all the instructions for whatever you're going to practise. That means not only the step-by-step guide for each posture, but also all the notes and recommendations for modifying or practising variations.

There are lots of different ways of practising the same posture, and you need to make sure that you're practising what's most appropriate for you. That might take a bit of trial and error, so look at the whole practice as a kind of experiment. Pay attention to the little changes you make and how it affects the feel of the posture.

Remember that the postures aren't a fixed shape that you're trying to achieve. The pictures are for reference, not because you're trying to put yourself into that exact shape. That's why there are also a lot of pictures included of ways of varying and modifying the postures if you need to. Don't worry about what it looks like, concentrate on how it feels. Remember that the variation that you can do today is enough.

WHEN YOU SHOULDN'T DO IT

In the instructions below for each of the individual postures there's a section headed "When you shouldn't do it." This is designed to give you a rough idea of whether it's a good idea for you to practise that particular posture right now or not. If you've read other yoga books, or looked at yoga websites online, you might have seen this information under the more medical sounding heading "Contraindications."

Above all, always check with your health care professional whether the course of activity you're intending to undertake is appropriate for you.

Some of the more traditional guides to yoga will tell you not to do certain yoga postures if you have a headache or diarrhoea or insomnia. This hasn't been included in the instructions below for several reasons.

Firstly, it should be obvious that you shouldn't engage in much potentially strenuous activity if you have a headache or diarrhoea. Anyone who has suffered from either knows that you don't want to be stuck in Downward dog when you feel like that. You might not be feeling your all-time best when you practise yoga - if you practise regularly, you'll know that sometimes you feel better than others. Some days you move more easily than others. However, make sure that you're in a physically fit state to perform the postures that you have decided to practise.

Secondly, it is very hard to say that complex conditions like insomnia, which have many contributing factors, will be made worse by one specific posture. There hasn't been any research done on these contraindications, and a lot of the time, they have been suggested by a teacher who simply has a certain feeling about the posture. That's not to say that practising yoga wouldn't influence something like insomnia, but it might have a different effect on different people for different kinds of insomnia.

Some of the traditional yoga guides also provide suggestions about whether you should practise yoga if you're menstruating, sometimes even flagging up postures that you should avoid. These suggestions haven't been included in the book, because there has been no good evidence to say that they have any value. What and how you practise during this time is a very individual choice and is best left to the individuals concerned. Practise if you feel like it, rest if you don't - and if you do practise you can do any of the postures.

PRACTISING WHEN PREGNANT

As above, you must always check with your health care professional whether the course of activity you're intending to undertake is appropriate for you, especially with pregnancy because of the potential for greater complications.

Advice is mixed about whether you should practise yoga when pregnant, especially in the first trimester: some say that no asana practice should be done, some say that the practice doesn't even need to be modified.

Remember that the first trimester is considered the riskiest in terms of miscarriage, so it is advisable not to over tax the body if it is already fatigued. If you're brand new to yoga, you're probably best seeking out a class that is designed especially for pregnancy, that way as your body changes over the months, you can adapt your practice with guidance from someone who has seen how you've been progressing.

NAMES OF POSTURES

When going through this book, you might come across postures that you've practised before but with a name that is different from the one in the book. Often, when new yoga systems get established and marketed, people try to come up with new English names for the postures to make them stand out. The names are only useful to help you identify the postures, and you don't need to try and remember them.

Where possible, the Sanskrit name of the posture has also been included. Almost all the postures end in the suffix "-asana." Asana is the Sanskrit for "posture" or "pose."

GET STARTED!

Start practising the postures - there's more details on how yoga works and its history at the back of the book. Everything makes more sense when you start trying things out.

WHAT YOU NEED

You don't need much to practise yoga. That's one of its great benefits. Most people like to practise on a yoga mat which can help keep your feet from slipping, but you don't need one. You could practise on the floor - although you'll probably prefer a carpeted one when you do postures that involve sitting, kneeling or lying on the floor.

Mats are quite good to give you a sense of place for your practice, something familiar and uniform, so I do recommend using one. You don't have to spend much on one, although you can if you want – high end mats are not cheap!

Having blocks when you're first starting out is quite useful - and there are many suggestions in the book of how you can use them. You can buy very inexpensive ones online, or you can use something equivalent you might have in your house. A big thick book works quite well, or better yet, a little box - as long as it's strong enough to press some of your bodyweight against.

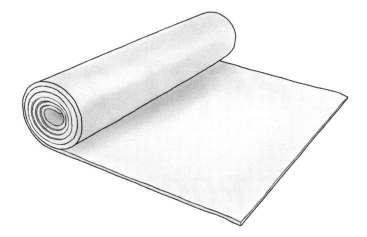

If your hamstrings are particularly tight, you might find using a strap is helpful - and the postures where you might need one are clear in the book. You can get yoga straps online, but really anything that's the same shape will work just as well. One of the best homemade options is to use the belt from a dressing gown if you happen to have one.

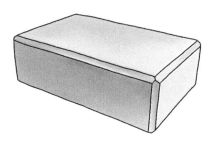

"Accomplishment in yoga is not achieved by wearing the apparel of a yogin, or by talking about it. Practice alone is the means to success."

HATHA YOGA PRADIPIKA

PART 2

THE POSTURES

CHAPTER 4

POSTURES TO GET YOURSELF STARTED

Everybody's got to start somewhere. Don't worry too much about where that starting point is. Often the biggest roadblock to getting going with something new is the feeling that you should be more capable at it, or that you're far behind everyone else. Sometimes that can make you feel that there's no point in even starting at all.

In yoga, everyone's on their own individual journey. It doesn't matter how many of the postures you can do, whether you find them challenging or not or whether you can stand on one leg without falling over a lot. What matters is that you meet yourself exactly where you are, without judgement.

Our modern culture runs its businesses on the principle that you are somehow lacking in something, that how you are right now is not enough. If only you could look a certain way, or have a special product, then you'd be happy. Yoga teaches the opposite. You have everything you need within you to find joy and be at peace with the world.

The following postures are a great way in. Not only do they lead on easily to the rest of the physical movements of the yoga asanas, but they are also a great way in to discover the rest of what yoga has to offer.

EASY POSE

Sukhasana

On one level, the whole experience of yoga can be encapsulated in this posture. You don't need to do complex postures to get the benefits of a yoga practice, you can do something as simple as this.

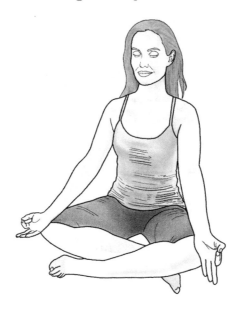

HOW TO DO IT

▷ Sit on the floor with legs crossed in front of you, so that the lower legs are touching, and the ankles are below the knees. Try to keep the spine straight so that you don't feel like you're slouching.

Although *Sukhasana* is often translated as "Easy pose" you might not find it that easy to begin with. If your lower back feels uncomfortable, try raising your hips up. Sit on a firm cushion, a bolster or even a yoga block if you have one.

If your knees hurt when you bend them, then only bend them as much as is comfortable. You can prop them up with cushions or fold them to different degrees to make sure they feel good. The idea is to sit in a comfortable position without excess pressure on any part of the body, especially the spine.

Easy pose is a great place to start a practice.

Sit with your eyes closed and try to come to a point of stillness. To begin with you might feel it's difficult to stay still. Don't worry if you fidget a bit and have to readjust to get yourself comfortable.

Breathe through your nose and check in with your body. Notice how your body feels today: are any parts of it sensitive or painful? Assess your energy levels: do you feel powered up and ready to go, or slow-moving and lethargic? Or something in between? And what direction are your thoughts headed in: notice how your mental state shifts and changes as you sit and breathe.

Sitting still and checking in is a great way to evaluate what kind of practice to do. That could also be all you do for the day! If you're short on time, sitting mindfully for a few minutes is a powerful way to start the day. If you feel strong and full of energy you could do a more dynamic practice, if you need to slow things down, do something restorative.

WHAT DOES IT DO?

This is a big question as far as Easy pose goes. It's a fundamental seated pose which you can use for breathing exercises or meditation. You can go to amazing places with both. If you practise Easy pose regularly, and start to associate it with your yoga practice, you might find that it automatically has a calming effect on you. You might find that the rest of the benefits of your yoga practice, the stress reduction and relaxation, will be associated with this posture.

WHEN YOU SHOULDN'T DO IT

Unless you're unable to sit up, you should be able to do some version of Easy pose. That might mean you have a lot of props supporting you. You can have cushions behind your back, you can lean against a wall. You can do a version of Easy pose sitting in a chair if sitting on the floor isn't an option at the moment.

CAT-COW

Bitilasana Marjaryasana

Cat-cow is a great way to warm up and get the spine moving at the beginning of a practice, but it can be done anytime. It's also an excellent movement to do after you've been sitting still for some time and can be used when you need a break from work.

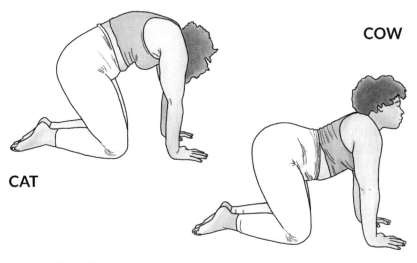

COW

CAT

HOW TO DO IT

▷ Start in all fours position with a neutral spine, with the knees under the hips and the hands under the shoulders.

▷ As you inhale, lift the chest up and draw the shoulder blades down while simultaneously trying to gently arch the lower spine. This is the cow part.

▷ As you exhale, round the spine, bring the chin to the chest and tuck the pelvis, so that the whole spine flexes. This is the cat position.

▷ Continue these movements, trying to synchronise the arching of the spine with the inhale and the rounding of the spine with the exhale.

▷ Finish after 5 or 6 rounds.

You don't have to do very big spine movements for this to be effective, in fact it's better to start small and go gently. If part of your spine feels like it doesn't move that easily, don't try and force it. Notice that some sections of your spine move through a much great range of motion than other parts.

WHAT DOES IT DO?

Cat-cow mobilises the spine, alternately stretching the front and the back of the body. It gives you greater awareness of your spine and how it moves, which can help you to become more attuned to your posture and habitual spine positions.

WHEN YOU SHOULDN'T DO IT

If your wrists or shoulders are injured and can't bear any body weight, this can be done in a seated position, either in Easy pose, or sitting on a chair, with your hands on your knees. Likewise, if you have a knee injury or arthritis in the knee and can't kneel.

Be careful if you have a back, neck or hip injury.

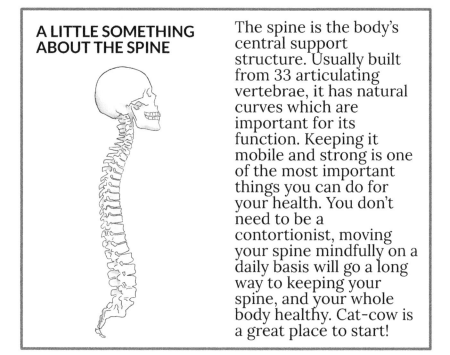

A LITTLE SOMETHING ABOUT THE SPINE

The spine is the body's central support structure. Usually built from 33 articulating vertebrae, it has natural curves which are important for its function. Keeping it mobile and strong is one of the most important things you can do for your health. You don't need to be a contortionist, moving your spine mindfully on a daily basis will go a long way to keeping your spine, and your whole body healthy. Cat-cow is a great place to start!

UNSTABLE ALL FOURS

In combination with Cat-cow, this posture - or pair of postures - provides a fantastic way to activate your core in preparation for any kind of movement, not just yoga practice.

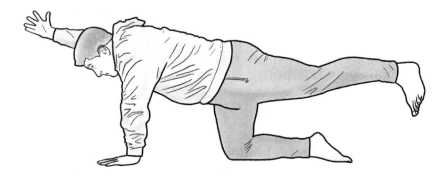

HOW TO DO IT

▷ Start in all fours position with a neutral spine, with the knees under the hips and the hands under the shoulders.

▷ Lift your right leg off the floor and extend it back behind you.

▷ Try to keep the spine neutral so that you're not arching the lower spine to lift the leg up.

▷ Shift the weight to your right hand and lift your left arm off the floor.

▷ Turn the palm to face inwards to externally rotate your shoulder.

▷ Stretch from the fingertips of the left hand to the toes of the right foot.

▷ Stay in the posture for about 30 seconds or several slow breaths.

▷ Repeat on the other side.

NOTES

Notice how much the rest of your body changes position when you lift the leg and the arm off the floor. Try to minimise the side-to-side movement of the body as much as possible.

TO CHALLENGE YOURSELF

You can add a movement to this to increase the core activation of the posture. Pressing firmly through the grounded hand and knee, round the spine and draw the knee of the lifted leg towards the forehead. At the same time, bend the elbow of the lifted arm and pull it back.

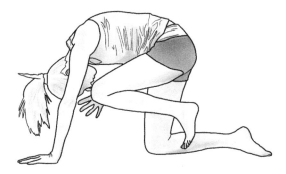

Don't worry if the forehead and the knee actually connect. Instead concentrate on getting as close as you can while keeping the rest of the body as still as possible. You can either hold the crunched positions or, like Cat-cow, you can link the movement to your breath for repetitions. Inhale as you extend, exhale as you compress.

WHAT DOES IT DO?

This posture is a great way of building core stability. Increased core strength and stability will improve your balance, protect your spine and keep you movable.

WHEN YOU SHOULDN'T DO IT

If your wrists or shoulders are injured and can't bear any body weight, or if you have a knee injury or arthritis in the knee and can't kneel, then avoid this posture.

THREAD THE NEEDLE

Combined with back bending postures, this pose is a great way to counteract all the time you might spend sitting down during the day.

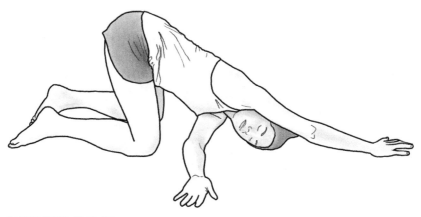

HOW TO DO IT

▷ Start in all fours position with a neutral spine, with the knees under the hips and the hands under the shoulders.

▷ As you inhale, lift your right arm up, stretch it up towards the ceiling and gently rotate your torso to the right.

▷ As you exhale, bring the right arm back down under your chest and through the gap between your left arm and your left leg to bring your arm and shoulder to the floor.

▷ Extend your left arm over your head and rest the side of your head on the floor.

▷ Stay in the posture for about 30 seconds or several slow breaths.

▷ Repeat on the other side.

NOTES

If you want to add movement to this, practise repetitions of lifting the arm up and threading it through on an inhale and an exhale. If you do this, you don't need to go to your maximum depth with each repetition - just work on rotating the spine and opening the shoulder, connecting the movement with the breath.

If your head doesn't reach the floor, you can support it with something like a cushion or a yoga block. Likewise, if your back feels uncomfortable, stay higher up and have some support underneath your head.

WHAT DOES IT DO?

As well as stretching the shoulder, this is a twist that focuses on mobilising the thoracic spine, the middle and least flexible part of the spine. This will have a knock-on effect on your posture and overall upper body flexibility.

WHEN YOU SHOULDN'T DO IT

If your wrists or shoulders are injured and can't bear any body weight, or if you have a knee injury or arthritis in the knee and can't kneel, then avoid this posture. Also avoid the posture if you have a spinal injury.

"Put your heart, mind, and soul into even your smallest acts. This is the secret of success."

SWAMI SIVANANDA

DIAMOND POSE

Vajrasana

This is a basic kneeling position. It can be used for meditation and breathing exercises, and it's also a good position to practice other physical movements. For instance, you can work on shoulder mobility (see below), neck stretches or wrist warm-ups. It can be practised at any point - at the beginning of a practice, or when you need to take a moment to rest during a sequence.

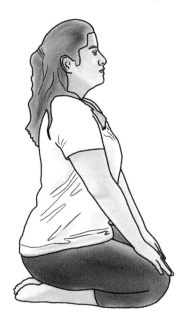

HOW TO DO IT

▷ Sit on your mat in a kneeling position.

▷ Try to keep your spine straight.

▷ Stay in the position for 30 seconds to a minute. You can of course stay longer if you're going to practise pranayama or meditation.

NOTES

Use as much support as you need to make sure that your hips, knees and ankles are comfortable. You can sit on a block to raise your hips up and put a rolled-up mat in between your calf muscle and hamstrings if necessary. If your ankles or the tops of your feet are uncomfortable, put extra padding underneath them.

If you find sitting in Diamond pose very easy, notice the different positions that your knees and ankles can be in. Touch your toes together and see if you can sit both with your heels touching and your heels apart. Notice the difference in sensation and effort depending on how you align your ankles.

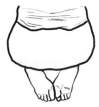 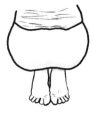

To stretch the soles of your feet, try tucking your toes underneath and sitting on your heels. If your toes hurt doing this, start by having the weight more forwards, and support yourself with your hands on the floor or blocks in front of you.

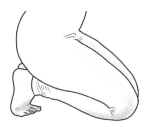

WHAT DOES IT DO?

Diamond pose gently stretches the thighs and ankles. By kneeling regularly and mindfully, you make sure that the knees will maintain the capacity to flex fully in a kneeling position.

WHEN YOU SHOULDN'T DO IT

If you have a serious knee or ankle injury, approach this posture very cautiously. Use as much support as necessary, but if it is still uncomfortable, avoid it until the injury has improved.

35

SHOULDER MOVEMENTS IN DIAMOND POSE

These are some ways of moving and stretching the shoulders that can be done as part of a warm-up while kneeling in *Vajrasana*, or incorporated into any of the postures where they seem like they might fit in. For instance, you could do Reverse prayer in Warrior 3, or in Intense side stretch pose (as is described in the instructions for the posture). Or you could try Cow face arms in Standing wide leg forward fold or Reverse warrior. You can also do them while standing in Mountain pose at the beginning of a practice.

▷ Eventually try to bring the palms of the hands together and draw the elbows towards each other, away from the sides of the body.

▷ Stay in the position for 30 seconds to a minute.

If you can't bring your hands together in a prayer position, you can try bringing your fists together instead, with the thumbs up and the little fingers down. If that is also too difficult, try grabbing the opposite elbows

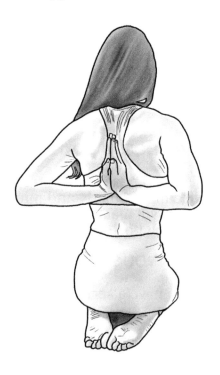

REVERSE PRAYER

▷ Bring your hands behind your back and touch the fingertips together.

▷ Once the fingertips are touching, start to push your hands up your back, in line with your spine, so that more of the front of the fingers are in contact.

behind your back. Both variations provide some of the same shoulder movement, but with reduced intensity.

WHAT DOES IT DO?

Reverse prayer particularly stretches the chest and front of the shoulders. It mobilises the shoulder, working the glenohumeral joint (where the arm bone joins the shoulder blade) into slight internal rotation, and stretches the wrists as well.

COW FACE ARMS

▷ Raise your right arm over your head and bend your elbow to bring your right hand towards the back of your neck.

▷ Bend your left elbow and reach your left hand up your back towards your right hand.

▷ If you can reach, clasp the hands together.

▷ Point your right elbow up towards the ceiling and straighten up the spine.

▷ Stay in the position for 30 seconds to a minute.

▷ Repeat on the other side.

If you can't reach your hands together, there are several options. You can use a belt, strap or towel - start with it in your top hand so that it hangs down for your bottom hand to reach. You can start to crawl your hands closer towards each other if you're using a prop like this, which will deepen the stretch. It's also fine to have your arms and hands in the general position, but without holding onto the hands.

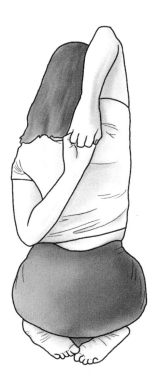

SHOULDER MOVEMENTS IN DIAMOND POSE CONTINUED

You might notice that you have different levels of flexibility on each side of the body, and this is normal. Everyone is a bit uneven. If you can reach your hands together on one side, but not the other, don't worry, and don't try to force both sides to be equal. Take your time. It's fine to use a strap on only one side if you need it.

WHAT DOES IT DO?

Cow face arms stretch the chest and latissimus muscles. It also can also provide a strong stretch for the triceps muscles. It can help improve shoulder mobility.

EAGLE ARMS

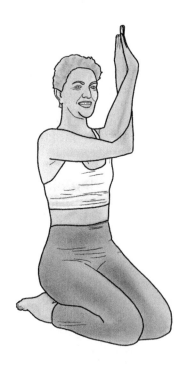

▷ As you inhale, bring both arms up over your head sideways.

▷ As you exhale, swing your right arm underneath the left arm and cross at the elbows.

▷ Turn your hands so that the thumbs are facing your face and the little fingers are facing away from you.

▷ Cross at the wrists to bring your palms together.

▷ Stay in the position for 30 seconds to a minute.

▷ Repeat on the other side.

If you can't reach the hands together, you can use a belt, strap or towel, although you don't need to - the action of moving your arms into the position works well on its own.

You can experiment with pulling the elbows up or down, towards or away from your chest, and notice the difference in sensation of what muscle groups are being stretched.

WHAT DOES IT DO?

Eagle arms stretch the back muscles, including the rhomboids, the lower trapezius and the teres major. It also helps to improve wrist and shoulder mobility.

WHEN YOU SHOULDN'T DO THEM

If you have serious neck or shoulder problems, approach any of these movements with caution. Both Reverse prayer and Cow face arms work the shoulder joint into internal rotation, which can be limited for many people. Never force the movements if they feel painful.

If you have serious wrist injuries, either modify or avoid Reverse prayer and Eagle arms.

LOW SQUAT

Malasana

Squatting as low as you can is a great test of lower body mobility. If you don't live in a culture where squatting is a part of everyday life, it's a good idea to do just that – make it part of your everyday life. It's a movement which has a great carryover benefit to so many kinds of physical activity.

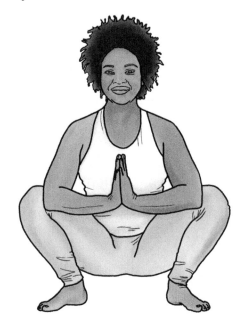

HOW TO DO IT

▷ Open your feet to about hip-width or slightly wider.

▷ You can turn your toes out slightly.

▷ Bend the knees and sit your hips down as low as possible.

▷ Bring your elbows inside your legs and press them against your inner knees or inner thighs.

▷ Bring your hands into a prayer position and resist your knees against the elbows.

▷ Lengthen your spine as much as possible.

▷ Stay in the position for 30 seconds to a minute.

NOTES

Notice whether the inner arches of your feet are rolled inwards, or the toes are excessively turned out. If this is the case and your heels are on the floor, you can try lifting them slightly to get the feet to point in the same direction as the knees and use some support under your heels.

Likewise, if your heels naturally lift off the floor when you squat down, you can put something underneath them, like a rolled-up mat or a folded blanket. This will give you something to press your heels against to help stretch the deep calf muscles and the Achilles tendon. Over a period of practising the posture you can experiment with lowering the support underneath your heels so that they get closer and closer to the floor. As you do this try to maintain a foot position so that the knees are pointing in the same direction as the toes.

Eventually you might find that you can get the heels down but keep on falling backwards. When that starts to happen, hold onto something (like a piece of furniture or a door frame), and gradually start to lessen the support so that you can balance freestanding. This may take some time, so be patient

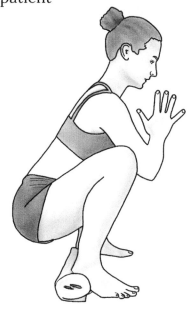

WHAT DOES IT DO?

Practising Low squat will improve mobility and stability in the ankles, knees, hips, pelvis, and spine. Squatting is also good for the digestive system.

WHEN NOT TO DO IT

If you have a lower back or knee injury, avoid the posture until the injury is resolved, or consider doing a very modified version with a lot of support under the hips - like a block or a low stool.

CHILDS' POSE

Balasana

Child's pose is a great way of starting or finishing a practice, or a way to take a break in between more challenging asanas. In the posture your spine is curved like that of a tiny baby, before the secondary curve in the lower spine starts to develop

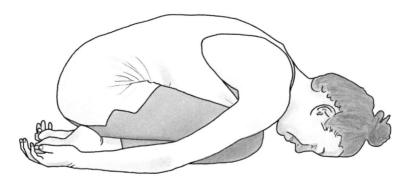

HOW TO DO IT

▷ Start in Diamond pose.

▷ Open your knees to about hip width apart.

▷ Bring your body down between your thighs and rest your head on the floor.

▷ Bring your arms alongside your legs with the palms facing up.

▷ Stay in the position for 30 seconds up to several minutes.

NOTES & ALTERNATIVES

You can also practise the posture with the arms extended out in front of you - either have the hands relaxed on the floor with the palms face down, or you can make it more active, and bring the palms together and stretch the fingertips away from the body.

You can use as much support as you need in this posture to make it more comfortable, especially if you are planning on staying in it for a little while. If you have difficulty reaching your head to rest on the floor, you can use a cushion or a bolster underneath it.

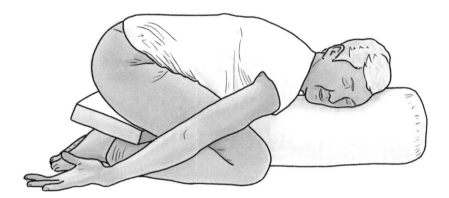

You can also put something behind the back of the knees to support the knee joint.

WHAT DOES IT DO?

Child's pose gives a gentle stretch to the hips, thighs and ankles, and to the back of the body and the front of the shoulders. If you have your arms out in front of you, your shoulders will be stretched in the overhead position, and if you're actively stretching the arms forward, then this will be intensified, as will the stretch of the spine.

Child's pose is a very relaxing posture, and in the right circumstances can help calm you down and relieve stress and tension.

WHEN NOT TO DO IT

If you have a knee or spinal injury, approach the posture with extreme caution, and avoid it completely unless you can practise a supported version completely pain-free.

CHAPTER 5

POSTURES FOR BOOSTING YOUR ENERGY

It's hard to think of a time when you didn't wish you had more energy. Yoga practice can help regulate your energy so that it'll be at a level that's more useful for your life. This means that you'll have more energy when you need it, and less when you don't. It means that you can use your energy to be more productive and effective at whatever you put your mind to.

One of the most energising and self-contained yoga practices you can learn to do is a sun salutation.

There are many different variations, but the most popular ones all follow a similar form, and you can change and vary them to suit your needs and circumstances. You can practise them slowly or quickly, and you can practise challenging versions of the postures or more accessible variations.

SUN SALUTATIONS
Surya Namaskar

A sun salutation is a series of postures practised in a sequence that flow into each other. All the different postures from the sun salutation can also be practised individually and can be used as part of any kind of practice.

Often the movements are linked to breath in a style of yoga that is called Vinyasa. Usually, an upwards movement or one that opens the front of the body is paired with an inhale, and a downwards movement or forward bend is paired with an exhale. (See Chapter 15 - Vinyasa)

Sun salutations are usually performed at the beginning of a practice. You could also do them during the middle part of the practice, while you're still doing standing postures (see Chapter 14 - Planning a practice), although most people like to use them to warm up. It's probably not best to do them at the end as they have a very stimulating effect on the nervous system and by the end, you usually want to calm things down.

In this book we'll look at three versions of Sun salutation. To help distinguish between them, we'll call them Surya Namaskar, Sun Salutation A and Sun Salutation B, even though *Surya namaskar* just translates as "sun salutation". Sun Salutation B is the most challenging version, but we'll see that it's possible to use variations of postures in all the different versions to make the movements accessible. Sun Salutation A and Sun Salutation B get their name from a popular style of yoga called Ashtanga Vinyasa Yoga.

HOW TO DO IT

If you're not sure how to do any of the individual postures, you can study the instructions in the rest of this chapter, which includes variations and advice on how to best practise them for your current physical state. It's a good idea to familiarise yourself with the different postures before you try and practise a whole Sun salutation. Go through each in turn and see how they feel in your body.

SURYA NAMASKAR

▷ Start in Mountain pose either with the arms by your sides, or the hands in front of the chest in a prayer position.

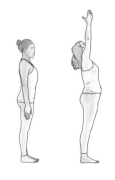

▷ Raise your arms over your head into Upwards arms pose and look at your thumbs.

▷ Hinge at the hips and bring your hands towards the floor into Forward fold. If you bend the knees at the beginning of the movement, it's often easier to make sure the hip hinges, otherwise you can end up rounding the spine.

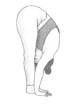

▷ Lift the upper body up and lengthen the spine into Half forward fold.

▷ Put the hands down flat on the mat, shoulder width apart, and step your right foot to the back of your mat. Put your right knee down onto the mat and come into Low lunge. You can keep your hands down or lift them up.

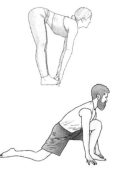

▷ Step your left foot to the back of your mat into Plank.

▷ Gently lower your knees down onto the mat, your chest and your chin, into Knees-chest-chin pose.

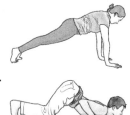

▷ Slide your body forward to bring your stomach onto the mat and, pressing through your hands, lift your chest up into Cobra pose.

▷ Curl your toes underneath so you can push through your feet, and simultaneously push through

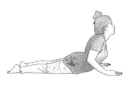

your arms to bring the hips back and up and your body into Downward dog.

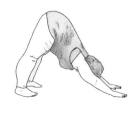

▷ Stay in Downward dog for about 30 seconds or several slow breaths through the nose.

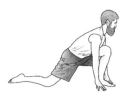

▷ Step your right foot forward in between your hands and put your left knee on the mat. Lift your arms up into Low lunge.

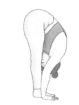

▷ Place your hands back on the mat either side of your right foot, shoulder width apart, and step your left foot forward to meet your right foot into Forward fold.

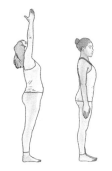

▷ Rise all the way up and bring the arms over the head into Upwards arms pose.

▷ Bring the arms back down by your side or in front of your chest in a prayer position for Mountain pose.

▷ Repeat the same sequence, this time stepping back and forward with the left foot.

SANSKRIT

The language of yoga is Sanskrit, a classical language of India. Almost all of the ancient texts that talk about yoga are written in Sanskrit. Although you don't need to know Sanskrit to be able to practise yoga postures, it's good to know some of the history of where they have come from.

I've tried where possible to put the name of the posture in Sanskrit. They also all have an English name as well, except for this one - Surya namaskar, which is pronouned *soorya namaskar*

SUN SALUTATION A

▷ Start in Mountain pose either with the arms by your sides, or the hands in front of the chest in a prayer position.

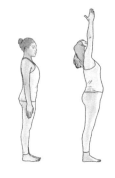

▷ Raise your arms over your head into Upwards arms pose and look at your thumbs.

▷ Hinge at the hips and bring your hands towards the floor into Forward fold. If you bend the knees at the beginning of the movement, it's often easier to make sure the hip hinges, otherwise you can end up rounding the spine.

▷ Lift the upper body up and lengthen the spine into Half forward fold.

▷ Step the right and then the left leg back into Plank.

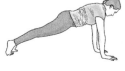

▷ Lower the body halfway down into Low-level plank.

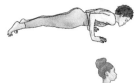

▷ Straighten the arms and simultaneously arch the spine into Upward dog, bringing the tops of the feet onto the floor.

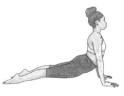

▷ Curl your toes underneath so you can push through your feet, and simultaneously push through your arms to bring the hips back and up and your body into Downward dog.

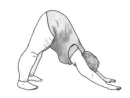

▷ Stay in Downward dog for about 30 seconds or several slow breaths through the nose.

▷ Step the right foot and then the

left foot forward in between the hands into Forward fold.

▷ Rise all the way up and bring the arms over the head into Upwards arms pose.

▷ Bring the arms back down by your side or in front of your chest in a prayer position for Mountain pose.

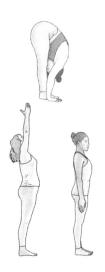

QUICK SUN SALUTATION MODIFICATIONS

One of the simplest ways to modify a sun salutation as a beginner, or if your wrists or shoulders hurt, is to swap out some of the more challenging postures for alternatives. The hardest part of the movement is often called the 'vinyasa', the combination of moving from Plank to Chaturanga to Upward dog and then Downward dog. If you find that really hard, start with these alternatives:

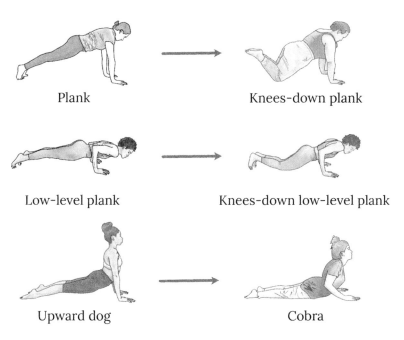

Plank   Knees-down plank

Low-level plank   Knees-down low-level plank

Upward dog   Cobra

SUN SALUTATION B

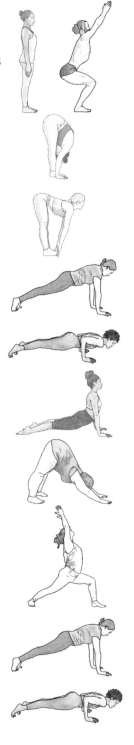

▷ Start in Mountain pose either with the arms by your sides, or the hands in front of the chest in a prayer position.

▷ Bend your knees and sweep your arms up over your head into Awkward pose.

▷ Hinge at the hips and bring your hands towards the floor into Forward fold.

▷ Lift the upper body up and lengthen the spine into Half forward fold.

▷ Step the right and then the left leg back into Plank.

▷ Lower the body halfway down into Low-level plank.

▷ Straighten the arms and simultaneously arch the spine into Upward dog, bringing the tops of the feet onto the floor.

▷ Curl your toes underneath so you can push through your feet, and simultaneously push through your arms to bring the hips back and up and your body into Downward dog.

▷ Step your right foot forward in between your hands, bend the front knee and lift the arms up over the head into Warrior 1.

▷ Bring the hands back down onto the mat and step your right leg back to Plank.

▷ Lower the body halfway down into Low-level plank.

▷ Straighten the arms and simultaneously arch the spine into Upward dog, bringing the tops of the feet onto the floor.

▷ Curl your toes underneath so you can push through your feet, and simultaneously push through your arms to bring the hips back and up and your body into Downward dog.

▷ Step your left foot forward in between your hands, bend the front knee and lift the arms up over the head into Warrior 1.

▷ Bring the hands back down onto the mat and step your right leg back to Plank.

▷ Lower the body halfway down into Low-level plank.

▷ Straighten the arms and simultaneously arch the spine into Upward dog, bringing the tops of the feet onto the floor.

▷ Curl your toes underneath so you can push through your feet, and simultaneously push through your arms to bring the hips back and up and your body into Downward dog.

▷ Stay in Downward dog for about 30 seconds or several slow breaths through the nose.

▷ Step the right foot and then the left foot forward in between the hands into Forward fold.

▷ Bend your knees and sweep your arms up over your head into Awkward pose.

▷ Bring the arms back down by your side or in front of your chest in a prayer position for Mountain pose.

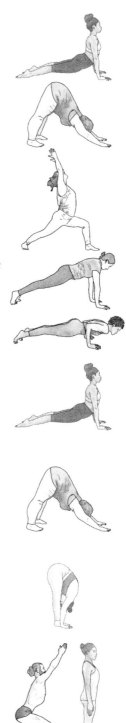

SUN SALUTATIONS

NOTES & ALTERNATIVES

In theory you can stay in any of the postures of each of the sequences for as long as you want. However, you'll definitely find it hard to hold postures like Low-level plank or Upward dog for very long!

Try to initiate each movement with an inhalation or exhalation. That means you might exhale down into Low-level plank and then inhale up into Cobra pose and exhale back and up into Downward dog. Then you'll only be in Low-level plank for a breath - but that will probably be enough!

If you practise a lot of Sun salutations, remember that repetitive movements should always be practised as mindfully as possible. Once you get familiar with the movements, it's easy to go into autopilot as you do them again and again. Try and avoid this as best you can: pay attention to how the movements feel, and do not exceed your capacity. If you start getting overly fatigued, you can always practise an easier variation of any of the postures in the sequence. That way you'll continue to get stronger and build up your endurance without experiencing overuse injuries.

A classic and challenging way of starting a strong vinyasa practice is to do 5 Sun salutation As and 5 Sun Salutation Bs.

TO MAKE THEM MORE ACCESSIBLE

If you find reaching the floor difficult in any of the sun salutation variations, try using some yoga blocks. You can have them ready at the front of the mat, so that they will be underneath your hands whenever your hands are on the floor. This can make the transitions of stepping forward and back much easier.

TO MAKE THEM MORE CHALLENGING

If you want to make Sun salutation A & B more energetic, instead of stepping forward and back, you can jump both legs at the same time. Eventually you jump back from the top of your mat to land straight in a Low-level plank, landing softly with control.

WHAT DO THEY DO?

Sun salutations do a lot! They stretch and strengthen almost every part of the body, mobilising all the major joints, including the spine. They're a great warm up for any physical activity, especially full body ones like martial arts, gymnastics or weight lifting. They're an amazing way to get your body moving in the morning.

Practising Sun salutation A or B will particularly strengthen the pectorals, deltoids and triceps - the pushing muscles at the front of the body - as well as the shoulders and core.

Have a look at what each individual posture does, and then combine it all to understand the incredible benefits of practising sun salutations!

WHEN YOU SHOULDN'T DO THEM

There are many different variations of all the postures involved in the sun salutations, so try and work out a sequence of postures to practice that works for you. It doesn't have to be the set pictured to be worthwhile doing. You can always also miss out parts if necessary - for instance the Low-level plank from Sun salutation A & B if you have a shoulder injury that feels worse when you do horizontal pressing movements.

However, if you have serious wrist or shoulder injuries, and can't do downward dog, it's best to practise other postures while the injury heals. Likewise, if you have spinal problems, be mindful of the movements from backward bends to forward bends - for instance Cobra or Upward dog to Downward dog. If you have a hip injury, be careful with Low lunge and Warrior 1.

MOUNTAIN POSE

Tadasana

Mountain pose is a whole practice in itself. It's the foundation of so many of the standing postures and although it seems very simple, you can easily get absorbed in the universe of details.

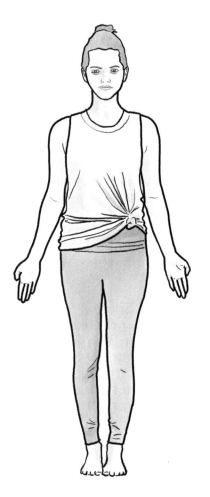

HOW TO DO IT

▷ Stand with your feet together. Many people like to have their big toes touching and the heels slightly apart.

▷ Balance your body weight evenly over the soles of the feet. Try lifting the toes off the floor and see how that helps you connect with the corners of the feet, and then gently spread and place the toes back down on the floor. Make sure your left side and right side are even.

▷ Try and find a position where your spine is under least tension: you're not overly arching the lower spine, or excessively rounding the upper spine. Notice if you're actively trying to do the opposite by tucking the tailbone or puffing up the chest. Instead try and bring your spine and hips into a neutral position.

▷ Allow your arms to hang by your sides, either with palms turned forwards, or palms facing the thighs.

▷ Notice where you're holding tension in the rest of your body, in particular relax your face, mouth and throat.

▷ Stay here for 1 minute, unless you're practising this as part of a set of Sun salutations.

NOTES

Foot position is very individual. You might find having your toes and heels touching feels great, or that you feel much more stable with your feet spaced. Experiment to find out what works best for you, and notice what happens at your knees, hips and spine when you change the position of your feet.

You can also practise this with your eyes closed. It's a great way to switch on your proprioception - your body's sensing system of where it is in space - and to turn your attention inwards at the beginning of a practice.

WHAT DOES IT DO?

Mountain pose helps you bring awareness to something that you might not normally think about: how you habitually stand. This can have a profound effect on improving your posture. Once you direct attention at something, then you can change it. In turn this can have an effect on conditions like flat feet and sciatica.

Mountain pose also acts as a foundation for all the other standing poses: try and bring the sense of balance and body awareness that the posture generates into everything else.

WHEN YOU SHOULDN'T DO IT

If you suffer from low blood pressure or dizziness, this can lead you to feel unstable, so make sure you have a supporting wall or chair nearby if you need it.

UPWARDS ARMS

Urdhva hastasana

This posture is rarely practised on its own. It is usually part of a Sun salutation.

Of course, it can be practised independently. A nice movement to do is to bring the arms up into *Urdhva hastasana* on an inhale and back down to *Tadasana* on an exhale and repeat several times to warm up the arms and shoulders.

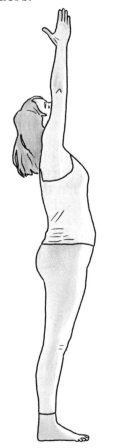

HOW TO DO IT

▷ Start in Mountain pose or standing with your arms by your sides.

▷ As you inhale, bring your arms out to the sides.

▷ As you start to lift your arms up, turn the palms to face the ceiling and continue to raise them up over your head.

▷ Bring your palms together and look up towards your thumbs without straining your neck.

▷ Lift the chest up while making sure you don't flare the rib cage or arch the lower spine.

NOTES & ALTERNATIVES

If your shoulders feel tight, you might find lifting them over your head makes you overly arch your lower spine. If this doesn't feel good, don't lift them as high. If your shoulders feel uncomfortable when you try to bring your palms together, then keep your hands apart.

You can also practice a variation of Upwards arms pose that is more of a backward bend. It's fine to practise this version, but try and make it a conscious choice. In other words, don't let restrictions in the shoulder joint force a backward bend.

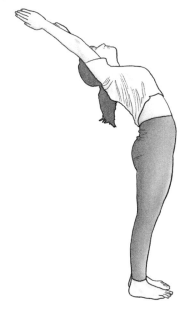

If you do practice this version, again you can keep the hands together or apart. Make sure you keep the legs, hips and abdominal muscles active to maintain stability, whilst continuously lifting the chest up towards the ceiling. This variation can be practiced both as part of a one-breath vinyasa, or as a posture in its own right that's held for several breaths.

WHAT DOES IT DO?

Upwards arms pose can help to release tension in the shoulder and upper back while stretching the front and sides of the body. It's great for keeping the shoulders mobile.

WHEN YOU SHOULDN'T DO IT

Avoid the movement if you have a neck or a shoulder injury that is made worse by raising the arms up.

FORWARD FOLD

Uttanasana

Developing the flexibility for a standing Forward fold can give you so many benefits. It might take time as well, so be patient with yourself. Don't worry about how far down you're going, instead pay attention to the sensation on the way down.

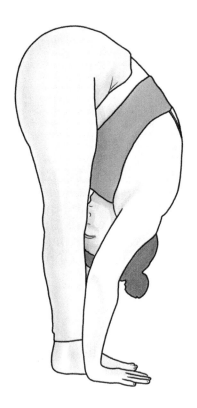

HOW TO DO IT

▷ If you're practising this at the beginning of a Sun salutation, you'll be in Upward arms pose, but you can also start in *Tadasana*.

▷ Bend forward at the waist, trying to hinge at the hip rather than rounding the spine, and bring your hands to the floor.

▷ Try to keep your legs as straight as possible.

▷ Line up your fingertips with the toes with your palms flat on the mat.

▷ Keep your quads (the front of the thigh muscle) engaged and lean your body weight forward so it is spread across the whole foot, rather than just in the heels.

▷ Allow your head to hang down, so your neck relaxes.

▷ Try to stretch your spine down.

▷ Stay in the posture for about 30 seconds or several slow breaths.

NOTES

Developing a hinge at the hips is the key to improving the Forward fold. If your hamstrings are very tight it can prevent the hip from flexing. Try bending the knees to get the hands down on the floor - to begin with don't worry if the fingers line up with the toes or not. Notice how bending the knees makes it a lot easier to bring the stomach closer to the thighs. Try and maintain the fold at the hips as you straighten the legs.

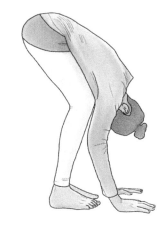

If the floor just feels too far away, even with the knees bent, then use some blocks under your hands. This will give you support, so you can experiment with stretching the back of the legs while trying to maintain the fold at the hips.

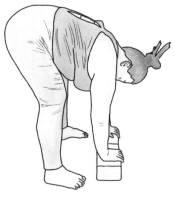

You might also find that opening the feet slightly makes the posture feel much more comfortable.

You can practise a variation of the pose where you grab the back of your heels, bringing the fingers under the feet, so you can pull on them to stretch the spine down. If you practise this variation, start with the knees bent.

WHAT DOES IT DO?

The standing Forward fold stretches the hamstrings, calves and back muscles.

It can also support a whole range of mental benefits, like helping to relieve stress, reduce anxiety and fatigue.

WHEN YOU SHOULDN'T DO IT

Avoid this posture if you have a lower back injury, sciatica or have an injured hamstring. Depending on how acute the hamstring injury might be, you can bend the knees to take the pressure off and still get some of the benefits of the forward bend.

HALF FORWARD FOLD

Ardha uttanasana

This posture is a powerful hamstring stretching pose which can be practised on its own, although it commonly forms part of the sequence of a Sun salutation. It's also a great way to find length in the upper body before going forward into a Forward fold.

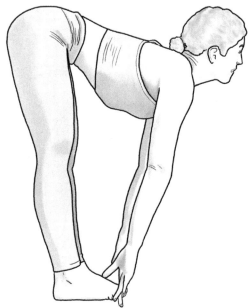

HOW TO DO IT

▷ From a standing Forward fold, push your hands or fingers against the floor and straighten the arms.

▷ As you inhale, arch the spine so the stomach comes away from the thighs and try to lengthen the torso forwards.

▷ Try and lengthen the lower abdomen.

▷ Lift the chest up and, being gentle with the neck, lift your head up and look forward.

▷ You can hold this for 30 seconds or several long slow breaths or continue onto the next part of the Sun salutation as you exhale.

NOTES & ALTERNATIVES

If you can't straighten the legs in a standing Forward fold yet, it is fine to practise the Half forward fold the same way, with the knees bent. This will make it much easier to lift the torso and feel the arch in the spine.

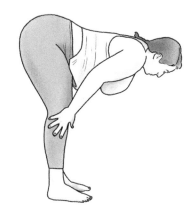

Alternatively, you can take the hands off the floor entirely and lift the torso much higher in order to get the spine straighter. You can place the hands on the thighs or the knees with the legs straight, or even slightly bent.

If you've been using blocks to assist with a Sun salutation, or you want to practise the posture and hold it for several breaths, have your hands on blocks for support. That way you'll find it much easier to lengthen the spine and stretch the front of the body, at the same time as getting the legs straight. You can lower the height of the blocks as your hamstrings become more flexible.

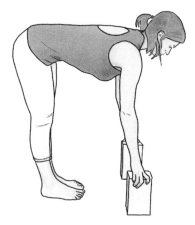

WHAT DOES IT DO?

The Half forward fold helps to activate the muscles on the back of the body, which can be good for your posture. With the legs straight, the posture stretches the hamstrings and calf muscles.

WHEN YOU SHOULDN'T DO IT

If you have a neck injury, don't lift the head up to look forward, keep the back of the neck long and look at the floor.

Just like with the standing Forward fold, avoid doing this if you have a lower back injury, sciatica or have an injured hamstring.

LOW LUNGE

Anjaneyasana

Most of us have tight or underused hip flexors from sitting on chairs so much, and the Low lunge is the antidote! This is a great posture to include as part of a workout recovery or to get moving in a slow and gentle way. It's a double-sided posture, so you need to make sure that you practise both sides. The below instructions are just for the right side.

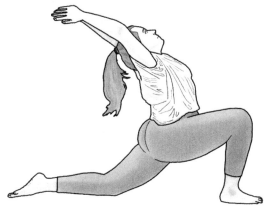

HOW TO DO IT

▷ Low lunge is easiest to enter from Downward dog or from a standing Forward fold.

▷ From Downward dog, step your right foot forward in between your hands and put your left knee down on the mat. From a standing Forward fold, step your left foot to the back of your mat and put the left knee down.

▷ Slide the left knee towards the back of your mat until you feel a stretch in the front on the left hip. Untuck the left toes and put the top of the left foot on the floor.

▷ As you inhale, lift your torso up and bring your arms up over your head.

▷ You can look straight ahead or bring your palms together and look at your thumbs by gently arching the spine into a backbend.

▷ Stay in the posture for several long slow breaths or about 30 seconds.

▷ Repeat on the other side.

NOTES & ALTERNATIVES

Keeping your hands shoulder width apart can feel much more comfortable than having palms together, so experiment to see what works best for you. If your neck hurts, keep the neck neutral and don't look at your thumbs.

Over time and with practise, you can develop the posture into more of a backbend, but take it slow to begin with, and focus on the sensation in the front of the hip of the leg that is going back.

If you want to hold the posture for longer than a few breaths, you can either practise it with the hands on the floor (or blocks) beside your front foot, or with your hands on the thigh of the front leg so that you can keep the spine more upright.

WHAT DOES IT DO

Low lunge stretches your quads and hip flexors. With the arms over the head, it stretches the shoulders, chest and abdominal muscles, and works on shoulder mobility in the overhead position. Stretching your hip flexors and keeping your hips moving can have a big impact on how your back feels.

WHEN YOU SHOULDN'T DO IT

If you have a knee injury or arthritis, and it hurts to put pressure on the knee, avoid the posture, unless pressure can be alleviated by using padding underneath the knee on the floor. Avoid the posture if you have a hip injury that is affected by the movement.

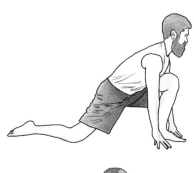

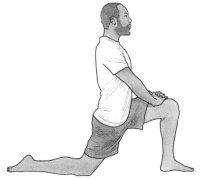

PLANK

Phalakasana

Plank pose is a fundamental strength building posture that works the whole body. Not everyone loves it to start with, but it's a building block to a stronger and more resilient body. And while it may look like a simple shape, the details will keep you working hard!

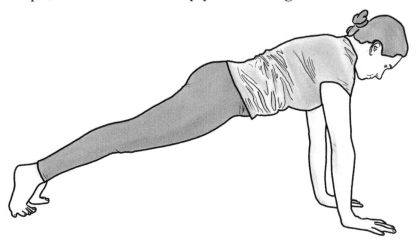

HOW TO DO IT

▷ You can either start in all fours or in Downward dog. If you start on all fours, step the right leg then the left leg back behind you. If you start in Downward dog, shift your body forward until the shoulders are over your wrists.

▷ Keep your arms and your legs straight - contract the triceps (the outer arms) and the quadriceps (the front of the thighs). Keep the toes curled underneath and press the heels to the back of the mat.

▷ Keep the neck and spine neutral. Try not to arch your spine or stick your hips up in the air.

▷ Try not to shrug the shoulder blades up by your ears, while simultaneously broadening them across your back.

▷ Hold for several long slow breaths or 30 seconds.

NOTES & ALTERNATIVES

If you find it very hard to hold for even a short time, you can start on all fours. Try to maintain a straight line from your knees to your shoulders, so that the shape resembles that of a plank.

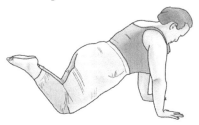

To progress, you can start by straightening one leg behind you. Hold for half the length of time on each leg and alternate the legs.

TO CHALLENGE YOURSELF

To develop endurance strength, you can try and hold Plank pose for time. Set yourself a target - for instance one minute - and see how many breaks you need to take to reach it. As you keep practising the posture, try and reduce the number of breaks. Once you reach the target without any breaks, set yourself a new target.

To develop weight-bearing strength, you can practise a 3-legged version of the posture. This means lifting either a leg or, which most people find much harder, an arm off the floor. Try and keep the rest of the body in the same position when you do it.

WHAT DOES IT DO?

Plank pose strengthens the arms, shoulders, wrists, and spine. It also activates and strengthens the core. You need to use the whole front of the body to keep yourself up there, and your abdominal muscles will prevent the spine from arching, so you'll definitely feel them working!

WHEN YOU SHOULDN'T DO IT

If you have a wrist injury or carpal tunnel syndrome, you can practise this on your forearms.

LOW-LEVEL PLANK

Chaturanga dandasana

Often called a "yoga push-up," Low-level plank is a part of many variations of Sun salutations or as part of the transition between postures. It can be practised in its own right and is a posture that even experienced yoga students find challenging.

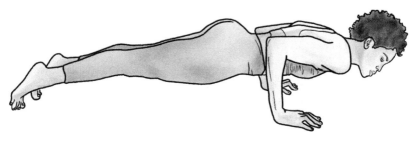

HOW TO DO IT

▷ Start in Plank pose.

▷ Try and maintain a strong plank position as you bend the elbows.

▷ As you exhale lower the body down until your chest is a few inches from the floor.

▷ Stay in control of the position of your elbows: don't flare them out wide or hug them in too tight to the side of the body.

▷ Maintain a strong activation of the core, so that the back doesn't arch, or the pelvis doesn't stick up high in the air (see below).

▷ You can hold Low-level plank for 30 seconds, or a few slow breaths. A common transition from the posture and one that is used in many Sun salutations is to bring the body forward into Upward dog on the next inhalation.

NOTES & ALTERNATIVES

Chaturanga is a difficult posture for many people, and it is worthwhile starting with a variation which places less stress on the shoulders.

From plank pose, if you put your knees on the floor and then perform the posture, this can provide enough support to allow you to work on keeping the spine straight, the core active and the shoulders stable throughout the movement. To begin with you can also lower down only a short distance.

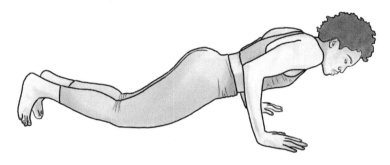

If you still find the posture too challenging with the knees on the floor, you can try raising your hands onto a higher surface. You can even start by standing up, facing a wall and just practise lowering towards and pushing away from the wall.

Always try to stay in control of the movement. In other words, don't let gravity take over so that you fall to the floor. Stop before you think your strength won't be able to keep you there. Likewise, try to maintain control over the position of the spine in the posture. Avoid arching the spine or sticking your hips up high in the air. If you find this keeps happening, then practise the pose with the knees on the floor and concentrate on how to maintain the pelvis and spinal alignment.

Avoid sticking your hips up...

...or arching your spine

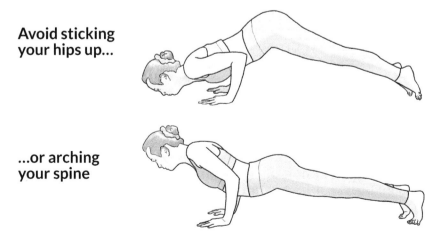

LOW-LEVEL PLANK CONTINUED

As the muscles, ligaments and tendons of the shoulder get stronger you can experiment with lowering down a little lower or taking one or both knees off the floor. Remember that your practice is always evolving. That might mean you start off practising a knees off the floor low version of chaturanga, but during the practice you change to a knees down, less deep version as your shoulders and arms get tired.

TO CHALLENGE YOURSELF

As you lower down, try to shift your whole body forward. You'll need to come onto the top of your toes to do this. This will mean that your shoulders will be quite far forward of your hand position, and your elbows will stack over your wrists. The further forward you bring your shoulders the more challenging the movement is, so always experiment slowly. Another way to challenge yourself is to practise a one-leg version of the pose. Make sure that your spine doesn't change position when you lift the foot off the floor.

WHAT DOES IT DO?

Low plank strengthens and stabilises the shoulder girdle as well as building strength in the core. The posture particularly works on the triceps, pectorals and deltoids.

WHEN YOU SHOULDN'T DO IT

Just like Plank or Knees-chest-chin pose, avoid this posture if you have a wrist injury or are suffering from carpal tunnel syndrome.

SPECIAL NOTE

If you find *chaturanga* challenging, try not to use Knees-chest-chin posture as an alternative. Make sure you understand the difference between the two postures, and consciously choose which one to practise. Practising a version of *chaturanga* with a lower load (knees down or less range of motion) will develop more strength overall in the long term.

KNEES-CHEST-CHIN

Ashtangasana

This is often used as one of the more traditional postures in a Sun salutation. You can practise it on its own, but it works very well as a transition between Plank and Cobra pose.

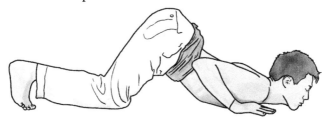

HOW TO DO IT

▷ Start in a Plank pose.

▷ As you exhale, lower your knees to the floor.

▷ While pushing through your hands, bend the elbows, arch the spine and bring the chest to the floor. Try and keep your elbows close to the sides of your body.

▷ Gently touch the chin down. Your shoulders will be more or less above your hands.

▷ If you're holding it for several breaths stay there, otherwise, on the inhale, slide your body forward so your hips come down to the floor so that you'll be ready for Cobra pose.

NOTES

If you don't think your chest will reach the floor, don't force it down. Get to where you get to in the lowering down phase and then slide forwards to bring the hips down if you're moving on to another posture.

WHAT DOES IT DO?

Knees-chest-chin pose improves spinal mobility and stretches the chest, which can help to prepare for backward bending postures. It helps develop some arm and shoulder strength – although not as much as Low-level plank and its variations.

COBRA POSE

Bhujangasana

Cobra pose is a great strength building backbend. It is a way of connecting with how the spine moves while having as much or as little support as you need from the ground and your arms.

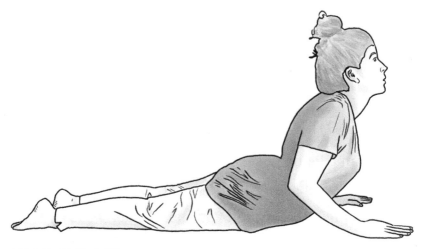

HOW TO DO IT

▷ Start lying on the floor face down. Place your palms directly underneath the shoulders.

▷ As you inhale, push down with your hands and start to straighten the elbows to lift the chest off the floor.

▷ Keep the elbows into the side of the body and pull them back and down to help draw the shoulder blades down the back and broaden the chest.

▷ Keep the hips on the floor - this will mean that the arms remain bent at about a 90-degree angle.

▷ Engage the glutes and leg muscles, at the same time lengthen the tailbone down to prevent the lower spine from overly arching.

▷ You can keep the neck neutral or gently arch it back in line with the rest of the spine.

▷ Stay in the posture for 30 seconds or several long slow breaths.

▷ Or if you're practising the posture as part of a Sun salutation, on the next exhale, curl the toes underneath and push the hips back and up into Downward dog.

NOTES

To lift the body off the floor in Cobra pose you need to use some arm strength. As the back muscles get stronger, you can gradually start to use less and less of the strength of the arms to keep yourself in the posture. You can even try and try and hover the hands off the floor - but remember to try and keep the legs down on the ground!

WHAT DOES IT DO?

Cobra pose increases the strength of the spinal muscles, particularly the big group that extends or backward bends the spine. In that way it improves spinal mobility, by giving you strength through a greater range of motion. This can improve posture over the long term and keeps the spine healthy.

It stretches the chest, shoulders and abdomen, and can stimulate the abdominal organs.

Cobra can boost your energy and help alleviate fatigue.

WHEN YOU SHOULDN'T DO IT & WHEN YOU SHOULD

If you have a wrist injury or carpal tunnel syndrome, practise Sphinx pose instead for some of the same benefits without the pressure in the wrist. If you have a back injury that means you can't extend the spine, avoid the posture until the injury has healed.

If you have a headache avoid backward bending postures.

*Often Cobra will be a good alternative to Upward dog.
If you're not feeling strong enough to hold yourself up in
Upward dog, practise Cobra pose instead.*

UPWARD DOG

Urdhva mukha svanasana

Upward dog is a big part of some variations of the Sun salutation sequences. Like Cobra pose, it helps to develop spine strength. However, Upward dog requires a great deal more strength overall to practise it in a comfortable way.

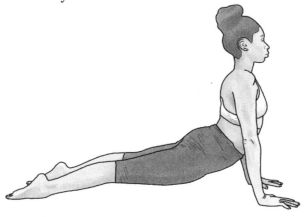

HOW TO DO IT

▷ Most of the time you'll probably come into this posture from Low-level plank as part of a Sun salutation, however it is possible to practise it on its own. If that's the case, start lying face down on the floor.

▷ From Low-level plank: as you inhale, straighten your arms and shift your body forward, so that you either roll over the top of the feet, or turn them over individually, so that the top of the foot is flat on the floor.

▷ If you're lying on the floor, have your hands under your shoulders, or a little below. Push strongly through your arms to straighten them and lift the torso up.

▷ Open the chest and arch the spine. You can keep the neck neutral or lift the head up and look up.

▷ Engage the leg muscles and the glutes. Lengthen the tailbone, so that the pelvis is neutral. Only the hands and the tops of the feet are on the floor - try and keep the hips off the floor.

▷ Try and stack the shoulders over the wrists and keep pushing strongly through the arms.

▷ Draw the shoulder blades down your back, to bring the shoulders away from your ears. It might feel as if you're trying to draw your chest and torso forwards by pulling with your arms.

▷ Hold the posture for 30 seconds or a few slow breaths.

Or if you're practising the posture as part of a Sun salutation, on the next exhale, curl the toes underneath and push the hips back and up into Downward dog. If you need to bring your thighs or hips down to the floor when you flip your feet over, that's ok. Then try to re-engage the thighs and lift them up off the floor.You don't need to bring your head up that far to look up towards the ceiling - always be gentle with your neck. Try and keep an even curve through the spine, including your neck. If your neck feels uncomfortable, keep the neck neutral and look straight ahead.

WHAT DOES IT DO?

This is a powerful back bending posture which strengthens the arms, wrists and all the back muscles. In fact, it strengthens the whole back of the body, which is often referred to as the "posterior chain". At the same time, it stretches the abdominal muscles, the chest and shoulders. Because of the action on the shoulders and scapula, this pose can have a beneficial effect on posture. Stretching the front of the body also stimulates the abdominal organs. Like Cobra pose, it can boost your energy and help alleviate fatigue.

WHEN YOU SHOULDN'T DO IT

If you have a wrist injury or carpal tunnel syndrome, practise Sphinx pose instead for some of the same benefit without the pressure in the wrist. If you have a back injury that means you can't extend the spine, avoid the posture until the injury has healed. If you have a headache avoid backward bending postures altogether.

AWKWARD POSE

Utkatasana

This is often referred to as chair pose, as it looks like you're trying to sit in a chair when you're doing the posture. Awkward pose strengthens your lower body and is used to initiate and finish the sequence of postures that make up Sun salutation B.

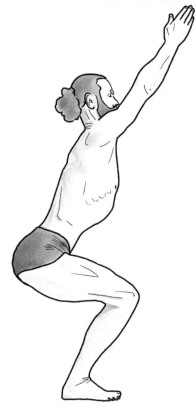

HOW TO DO IT

▷ Start in Mountain pose.

▷ Bend your knees deeply to try and bring your thighs as close to parallel to the floor as you can.

▷ Simultaneously sweep your arms up over your head and bring the hands into a prayer position or keep them shoulder width apart. Look up at the hands without straining the neck.

▷ Make sure that you're not gripping the floor with the toes and try to shift your bodyweight back to the heels.

▷ Hold the posture for 30 seconds or several long slow breaths.

NOTES & ALTERNATIVES

These instructions are just the very basics. There are lots of different variations of Awkward pose, all based on these same principles.

You can have the feet apart, especially if it is uncomfortable to keep them together. If the feet are apart, keep the knees apart as well and try to maintain the same distance between knees and feet throughout the posture.

If you have trouble lifting the arms up over the head, you can have them lower down either parallel to the floor, alongside the torso, or with the hands in prayer position in front of the chest.

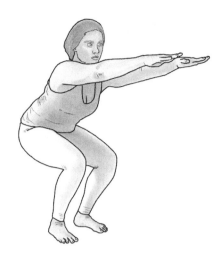

It's also possible to practice a more quad-dominant version of the posture, by lifting the torso more upright, and allowing the knees to travel forward in space. This will mean that they might go beyond the toes, so be mindful of how your knees feel if you perform this movement.

As you bend the knees, also notice what is happening at your feet and ankles in all the different Awkward pose variations. You might find the feet want to pronate or supinate (the ankle rolls in or out), or that the feet try to turn out. Try your best to keep the ankles neutral, and the feet to point in the same direction from beginning to end. In other words, don't go too low too quickly. Work on developing strength as you increase the depth of the movement.

WHAT DOES IT DO?

Awkward pose engages and strengthens the muscles of your lower body: the legs and hips. It also engages the core so that you stay stable and balanced. Depending on where you position your arms, it can also stretch the shoulders.

As a standing squat, Awkward pose is a posture that matches some of the everyday movements you make, like sitting down and getting up out of a chair, making it functionally useful.

WHEN YOU SHOULDN'T DO IT?

If you have a hip, knee, ankle or back injury, avoid this posture until the injury has sufficiently recovered. You can always practise the posture using support, such as a chair or the wall, and limit the depth to which you lower the hips.

WARRIOR 1

Virabhadrasana 1

Warrior 1 is a powerful lunging posture. It is often used in one of the more challenging variations of a Sun salutation, and it is a great way of warming up and strengthening the lower body ready for any kind of practice or workout.

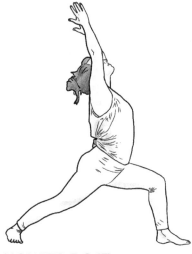

HOW TO DO IT

▷ If you practise this posture as part of a Sun salutation, you'll enter it from Downward dog: step your right leg forward between your hands, bend the right knee and come up into the posture with your arms over the head.

▷ Otherwise, start in Mountain pose. Step your feet out until they are 3 and half or 4 feet apart.

▷ Turn your left foot in so it's at a 45-degree angle at the same time as turning your right foot out 90 degrees so it points straight ahead. Try to keep the heels in one line.

▷ Bring your arms over your head and your palms together.

▷ Bend your right knee until your right thigh is parallel to the floor.

▷ Arch your torso up and back to look up at your thumbs, without overly straining the neck.

▷ Try and gently push your left hip forward to square the hips, while keeping the left heel on the ground.

▷ Hold the posture for 30 seconds or several long slow breaths.

▷ Repeat on the other side.

NOTES & ALTERNATIVES

If you practise this posture as part of a Sun salutation, you'll leave the posture by bringing your hands either side of your front foot and stepping the leg back to a Plank or Low-level plank.

For a posture that is often repeated many times as part of a set of Sun salutations, Warrior 1 is a surprisingly challenging posture. If your ankles or hips don't like the movement very much, try and practise it with the feet set wider apart. In other words, rather than having the heels on one line, set them hip distance apart. (See 'A short note on feet' after Side angle). Taking a shorter stance - 3 and half rather than 4 feet - can also make the back leg feel more comfortable.

If the shoulders feel uncomfortable, don't bring the palms together, instead keep them shoulder width apart. If raising them is difficult, you can keep them in a prayer position in front of your chest. If your neck hurts to look up at the thumbs, keep it neutral and look straight ahead instead.

A great alternative to Warrior 1 is High lunge. The form of the posture is very similar to Warrior 1, the main difference is that the back heel is lifted. It can be used as a replacement for Warrior 1 in a Sun salutation, or as

part of any kind of practice. Like Warrior 1, you can have the palms together or the arms apart, you can look up towards your hands or look straight ahead.

WHAT DOES IT DO?

Warrior 1 particularly stretches and strengthens the legs and hips. In fact, it stretches the whole front of the body as well as the chest and shoulders. It improves your balance and focus and can help to create a sense of strength and confidence.

WHEN YOU SHOULDN'T DO IT

Avoid or modify this posture if you have a leg, hip, knee or shoulder injury. This posture is also usually not recommended if you have high blood pressure or heart problems.

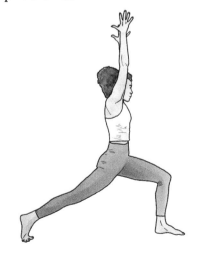

DOWNWARD DOG

Adho mukha svanasana

Downward dog is one of the most iconic and commonly practised yoga postures. It's often one of the first yoga postures you'll learn and if you practise Vinyasa yoga which includes Sun salutations, you'll do it quite a lot during the course of one practice.

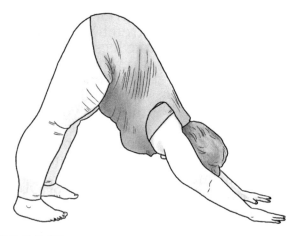

HOW TO DO IT

▷ As part of a Sun salutation, you'll come into the posture from either Cobra pose or Upward dog.

▷ Otherwise start on all fours, with a slightly longer stance. If your knees are under your hips, then bring the hands slightly forward from under your shoulders.

▷ Curl the toes so you can push through the feet and bring your hips up and back.

▷ Try to straighten the legs and contract the quadriceps (front of the thigh muscle).

▷ Shift the body weight towards the heels of the feet and try to bring them towards the mat.

▷ Externally rotate the shoulders while pressing the index finger side of the palm against the floor.

▷ Have your hands roughly shoulder width, and your feet roughly hip width.

- ▷ Try and keep the feet parallel so that the heels aren't pointing inwards, and keep the knees pointing forward, so that the thighs aren't rotating outwards.

- ▷ Hold the posture for up to a minute.

NOTES & ALTERNATIVES

Sometimes yoga teachers refer to this as a "resting posture" but for most people it is far from that. You might find it very challenging to hold your arms over your head whilst pressing your body away from the floor.

To begin with, you might find it easier to keep the knees bent and the heels lifted off the floor, especially if you have tight hamstrings. By bending the knees, you can untuck the pelvis so that you feel like you can begin to lengthen the lower spine. Even if the heels are off the floor, still try to shift the weight back to the heels, so your body weight is more evenly distributed between the hands and the feet.

Eventually you may be able to get the legs straight and the heels on the floor without the lower spine rounding, but don't worry if that takes some time, or even if it doesn't feel like it's happening. It's fine to keep the knees bent during the posture, because there are plenty of other ways to stretch your hamstrings!

If your shoulders or upper back feels tight, try practising the posture with your hands on blocks. This also helps for tight hamstrings. Using blocks underneath your hands can also make the transitions into and out of Downward dog from lunging postures much more accessible.

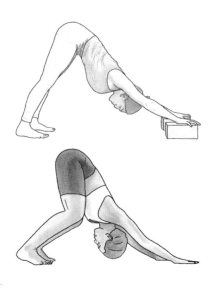

DOWNWARD DOG CONTINUED

TO CHALLENGE YOURSELF

Try lifting one leg off the floor into a 3-leg Downward dog. You can add an extra hip and side stretch by bending the knee of the top leg and turning the hip out.

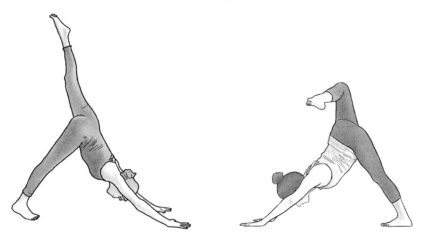

WHAT DOES IT DO?

Downward dog stretches the calf muscles and hamstrings. It strengthens the arms and shoulders in the overhead position. It also works to extend the spine on its axis - in other words it lengthens and decompresses the spine.

The posture also acts as a mild inversion because it brings your heart above your head and gives some of the positive benefits to the nervous system and cardiovascular system that inversions provide.

WHEN YOU SHOULDN'T DO IT

If you have a wrist injury, be careful when practising Downward dog - you can try placing a rolled-up towel underneath your palms on the wrist side, which might take some of the pressure off.

Likewise, if you have a shoulder injury, approach the posture cautiously.

CHAPTER 6
POSTURES THAT KEEP YOU GROUNDED

Keeping the lower body strong and flexible is the key to feeling mobile and able to navigate your world with ease. This set of postures does exactly that, working on creating stability while the legs are set wide apart. This will keep you feeling strong with your feet firmly planted on the ground.

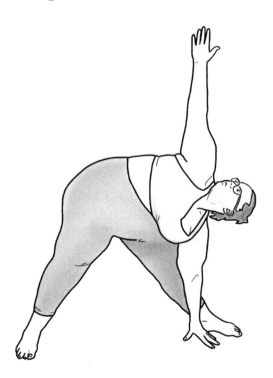

WARRIOR 2

Virabhadrasana 2

Warrior 2 is like Warrior 1 in the sense that it's a wide lunge. However, the difference in the position of the hips, feet and arms changes the feel of the whole posture.

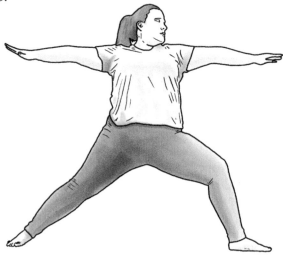

HOW TO DO IT

▷ Start in Mountain pose.

▷ Step your feet apart about 4 feet. Turn your right foot out 90 degrees so it points forward and turn your left foot in only slightly. Try and keep your heels in one line.

▷ As you inhale, bring your arms up parallel to the floor with your palms facing down.

▷ As you exhale, bend your right knee to bring your right shin perpendicular to the floor. If you can, try to sit the hips down low enough to bring the right thigh parallel to the floor.

▷ Try and keep your right knee stacked over your right heel, so that your bodyweight doesn't push forward into your right toes.

▷ Try and keep the spine straight in the centre, the shoulders stacked above the hips.

▷ Turn your head and look over the right hand.

▷ Hold the posture for up to a minute or several long slow breaths.

▷ Repeat on the other side.

NOTES

The distance between the feet along the length of the mat will determine how low you can bring the hips down. If your hips feel really tight, don't go too wide with the stance.

However, if your feet are too close together, you might find that the knee of your front leg pushes forward over the toes, and you should then open your feet wider. Remember that the wider the stance, generally the more challenging the posture will be.

Try not to let the front knee roll inwards: aim to point the knee over the front toes. If you find this difficult, try taking the feet wider from side to side. So instead of having the heels in one line, keep them about hip width apart.

WHAT DOES IT DO?

Warrior 2 activates the muscles of the arms, legs, shoulders, and back, while stretching the legs and hips, particularly the inner thighs. It can help relieve sciatica, flat feet and backache.

Like Warrior 1, it improves your balance and focus and can help to create a sense of strength and confidence. This in turn can increase your stamina as you stretch and strengthen the lower body.

WHEN YOU SHOULDN'T DO IT

Avoid or modify this posture if you have a leg, hip, knee or shoulder injury. This posture is also usually not recommended if you have high blood pressure or heart problems.

REVERSE WARRIOR

Viparita virabhadrasana

Reverse warrior is a great posture to practise straight after Warrior 2 as your body will be in the right position to go right into it. It's expressive and opens up the side of the body from a position of grounded strength.

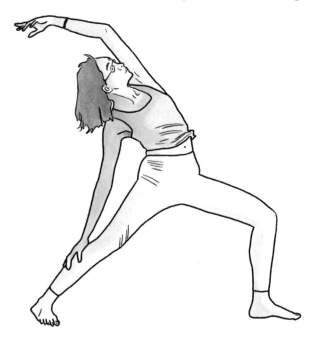

HOW TO DO IT

▷ Start in Warrior 2 pose (with the right knee bent).

▷ As you inhale, turn your right palm up to face the ceiling and raise the arm up towards the ceiling.

▷ Bring your left hand onto your left thigh.

▷ Lengthen the right side of your body and look at your right hand.

▷ As you lift your right arm up and back, stay strong through the legs and keep the hips in the same position.

▷ Hold the posture for 30 seconds or several long slow breaths.

▷ Repeat on the other side.

NOTES

Aim to create a nice even stretch down the side of the body. That means you don't need to go back deeply in the posture. Think of using your core muscles to support the torso.

If it hurts to bring your arm over your head, you can practise the same movement with the hands in front of your chest in a prayer position, and if your neck feels sensitive, keep it neutral and look straight ahead.

TO CHALLENGE YOURSELF

Try lifting the front heel off the floor so you're on your tiptoes to get the calf muscle to fire up!

What does it do?

Like Warrior 2, Reverse warrior builds strength and flexibility in the lower body. With the additional arm and spine movement, the posture stretches the sides of the body and the shoulders and strengthens the obliques. It also helps to improve mobility of the spine and can energise the whole body.

WHEN YOU SHOULDN'T DO IT

Avoid or modify this posture if you have a leg, hip, knee or shoulder injury. Also avoid the posture if you have a back or spine injury that prevents side flexion. This posture is also usually not recommended if you have high blood pressure or heart problems.

"Without understanding yourself, what is the use of trying to understand the world?"

RAMANA MAHARSHI

TRIANGLE POSE

Trikonasana

Triangle pose is a classic yoga posture that looks deceptively simple. The details can be harder than they look! It's a great pose to start to bring awareness to the different directions that the hip can move in, to being able to move the hips and the spine separately and to bring a sense of expansiveness to the whole body.

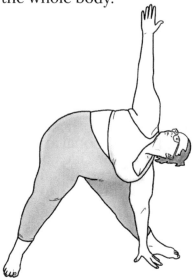

HOW TO DO IT

▷ Start in Mountain pose.

▷ Step your feet about 3-4 feet apart. Turn your right foot out 90 degrees so it points forward and turn your left foot in only slightly. Try to keep your heels in one line.

▷ As you inhale, raise both arms up parallel to the floor, palms facing out.

▷ As you exhale, reach your right arm forward over your right leg, bending at the right hip.

▷ Lengthen both sides of the body and bring the right hand down towards the floor, and the left arm up towards the ceiling.

▷ Keep your bodyweight spread evenly through both feet, grounding through the outer edge of the back heel.

▷ Turn your head and look up towards your left hand.

▷ Hold the posture for 30 seconds or several long slow breaths.

▷ Come out of the posture by bringing the spine back up to the centre.

▷ Repeat on the other side.

NOTES

To begin with, don't bring your bottom hand too low. Start with it resting on the shin or the ankle of the front leg, or you can use a block if you need a more stable support. Take your time to bring the hand lower down the leg or to the floor. If you bring the hand too low too quickly, the movement might come from the spine, rather than the hips. In other words, rather than folding at the front hip, the spine will just side bend. Try to notice where you feel sensation as you perform the movement.

Try not to lean the body forwards to bring the hand lower either - triangle isn't a forward fold - if you find it hard not to, then keep the bottom hand higher up.

You can also keep a tiny bend in the front leg, that way you will engage the hamstring of the front leg which will help to keep the knee more stable.

If your neck feels sensitive, keep the neck neutral and just look straight out to the side or at the ground to keep it in a comfortable position.

WHAT DOES IT DO?

Triangle pose stretches and strengthens the legs and hips, particularly the front leg. It also stretches and strengthens the muscles of the side of the body and activates the core.

At the same time as it stimulates the nervous system, it can also be a calming posture and help to reduce stress and anxiety.

WHEN YOU SHOULDN'T DO IT

If you have a leg, hip or ankle injury, avoid this posture, or be mindful of the depth you go into it. You can always practise it with the lower hand on the thigh above the knee and move through a more limited range of motion. If you have a neck injury, keep the neck neutral.

If you are having serious balance issues, you can practise this posture against a wall, so that you have much more support.

REVOLVED TRIANGLE

Parivrtta trikonasana

Revolved triangle is a powerful spine twisting pose that relies on the strong support of the legs and hips.

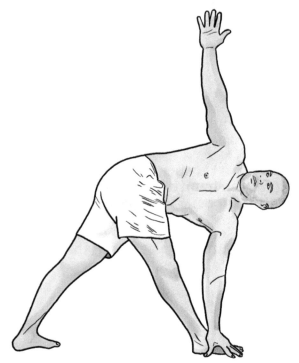

HOW TO DO IT

▷ Start in Mountain pose.

▷ Put your hands on your hips and step your left foot back about 3 to 3 and half feet.

▷ Turn your left foot out to a 45-degree angle so you can keep your back heel on the floor. Try to keep the heels in one line.

▷ Raise your left arm up so it's parallel to the floor.

▷ Try and keep both hips facing forward - notice that with your back leg stepped back, the pelvis might have changed position.

▷ Stretch your left arm forward to fold at the hips and

bring your body down. Lengthen both sides of the body evenly and try to prevent the spine from forward bending.

▷ Reach your left hand towards the floor on the outside of your right foot.

▷ Rotate your torso to the right and stretch your right arm up towards the ceiling.

▷ Turn your head and look up at your right hand.

▷ Hold the posture for 30 seconds or several long slow breaths.

▷ Repeat on the other side.

NOTES & ALTERNATIVES

Just like in Triangle pose, the key to this posture is not to go too low too quickly with the bottom arm. Start with the hand on a block in its highest position. If you don't have a block, you can put your hand on your front leg - on the shin or even higher up above the knee, depending on your flexibility. A block will usually make you feel more stable as you have three points of contact with the floor. As your practice develops, you can change the orientation of the block to bring your hand lower down and closer to the floor.

Try to make sure that the twist comes from the spine - think of the chest moving, rather than only the top shoulder. In other words, don't try and bring the top hand as far back as possible for the twist - see if you can get both shoulders to move equally. If you find the twist particularly challenging, start with the block on the inside of the front foot.

If the shoulder of the top arm feels very uncomfortable, keep the hand on the hip. That way you can also feel how much of the movement of the twist is coming from the spine as opposed to

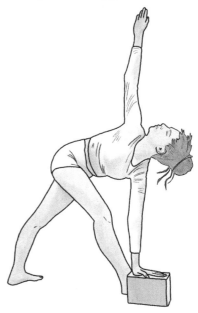

the hips. Don't force the neck round to look at the top hand. If the movement hurts your neck, then look at the ground or out to the side, keeping the neck neutral.

As with all these long stance postures, if you find the position of the hips very challenging and uncomfortable, practise it with the feet set wider side to side. In other words, rather than having the heels on one line, set them hip distance apart (see 'A short note on feet').

WHAT DOES IT DO?

Revolved triangle stretches the hamstrings, calves and hip muscles. It also works to strengthen the hip and leg muscles to keep the base of the spine stable for the twist.

Twisting postures stretch and strengthen the abdominal muscles and improve the mobility of the spine. In that respect they can help to relieve mild back pain. They also stimulate the abdominal organs and digestive system.

WHEN YOU SHOULDN'T DO IT

If you have a neck or a spine injury, lower back or sacroiliac joint pain, then avoid this posture.

If you are having serious balance issues, you can practise this posture next to a wall, so that if you were to lean against it, your back would be supported by the wall. In other words, twist away from the wall.

AGNI

In yoga and Ayurveda (an ancient alternative medicine system), the term *agni* is used in the sense of digestion of food and metabolic products. It is the energy that digests, absorbs and assimilates the food that you eat. Twisting postures are said to increase *agni* in the body, leading to more efficient metabolism and a stronger digestive system.

SIDE ANGLE

Utthita parsvakonasana

Side angle is a great posture to stretch the side of the body in one long connected chain. It requires a great deal of range of motion in the hip joint for the most challenging version, but there are always ways of making it more accessible. And of course, practising it regularly will definitely improve your hip flexibility!

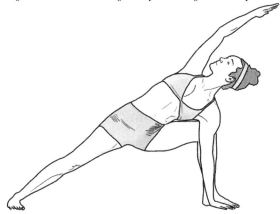

HOW TO DO IT

▷ Start in Warrior 2 with your right foot forward (see above).

▷ Bring your right hand down inside your right foot and put your hand or your fingertips on the floor.

▷ Extend your left arm up towards the ceiling and then reach it over your head, turning the palm to face the floor to externally rotate the shoulder. The bicep of your left arm will be close to your left ear.

▷ Lengthen the entire left side of your body by reaching forward through your fingertips while simultaneously pressing the outer edge of your left foot against the floor.

▷ Press your right knee and your right arm together and rotate your torso to the left as if trying to turn your chest up towards the ceiling.

SIDE ANGLE CONTINUED

▷ Turn your head to look at your left arm and then up to your left hand, without straining the neck.

▷ Hold the posture for 30 seconds or several long slow breaths.

▷ Repeat on the other side.

NOTES & ALTERNATIVES

With all the postures you're not trying to make a particular shape, but rather feel the effects of doing the movement and notice the physical and mental sensations that arise. This is especially true of Side angle. For many people it can be incredibly challenging to bring the hand to touch the floor and stay in the posture comfortably. Pay attention to how the front hip feels - if it feels like there's a lot of pressure there because the thigh is so close to the torso, then use a block underneath your hand. Don't force yourself into a position just for the sake of it.

If a block is still too low, or to keep the torso even higher, you can practise the posture with the forearm on the thigh for support.

If your shoulder feels uncomfortable bringing your arm over your head, then you can keep your arm resting along your side. If your neck hurts, keep the neck neutral and don't turn your head.

Keeping the back heel grounded on the floor as you go into the posture can be challenging. If this is the case, you can try practising the posture with your back heel against a wall. As you bend the front leg and bring the

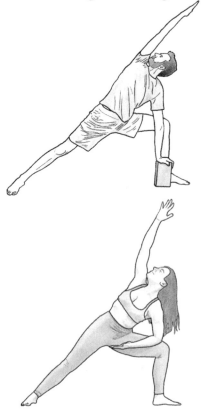

body down, use the wall as a reference by pressing your heel against it like you're trying to push it away. You might find that you don't go as low with the front leg or the torso, but that's fine.

WHAT DOES IT DO?

Side angle stretches the legs, particularly the inner thighs, the hips and the whole side of the body. It also works to strengthen the legs and hips. With the arm reaching beyond the head, the posture will stretch the shoulders, and open the chest.

By compressing one side and stretching the other side of the body, you stimulate the abdominal organs and digestive system.

Just like Warrior 2, this is a challenging lunging posture, and holding it will increase your stamina and your capacity to do all the other standing postures.

WHEN YOU SHOULDN'T DO IT

Avoid or modify this posture if you have a leg, hip, knee or shoulder injury. This posture is also usually not recommended if you have either high or low blood pressure.

A SHORT NOTE ON FEET

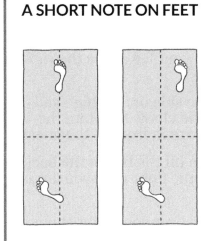

If you find any of the wide stance positions in this section challenging or a bit unstable, you can modify the position of the feet from the picture on the left, to the picture on the right, so that the heels are placed hip width across the width of the mat. This applies to all the postures in this section (apart from Standing wide leg forward fold), as well as Warrior 1.

REVOLVED SIDE ANGLE

Parivrtta parsvakonasana

This posture combines the power of a spine twist with the strength and stamina of a lunge.

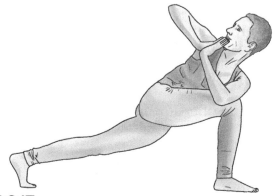

HOW TO DO IT

▷ Start on all fours or in Downward dog.

▷ Step your right foot forward in between your hands, and if your back knee is up off the floor, bring it down.

▷ Lift your torso up, so that the spine is upright and you're in a version of a Low lunge.

▷ Bring the hands in front of the chest in a prayer position with the elbows out wide to the sides.

▷ Rotate your torso to the right and try to reach your left elbow to the outside of your leg above the right knee.

▷ Push your elbow against the side of the thigh and push the leg back against the elbow to rotate the torso more until the hands are in front of the chest.

▷ Curl the back toes and push off the ball of the back foot to lift the left knee off the floor until you are in a lunge.

▷ Look up towards the ceiling over your right shoulder.

▷ Hold the posture for 30 seconds or several long slow breaths. Repeat on the other side.

To begin with it can be easier to work on the twist without lifting the back knee off the floor. Once you're comfortable with the twist, then work on raising yourself up into a lunge. Don't force the twist: if the hands aren't in front of the chest, it doesn't matter. Instead, think of lengthening the spine on its axis as you rotate it.

If you feel that the twist is very restricted, instead of trying to bring the elbow round the side of the leg, place your hand on the floor or on a block in line with the front foot, and lift the opposite arm up towards the ceiling to create the twist. You can keep the back knee down or curl the toes and lift it up into a lunge.

If your neck feels uncomfortable, keep it in a neutral position, rather than turning the head to look up at the top hand.

TO CHALLENGE YOURSELF

If you find the posture quite comfortable, instead of having the hands in a prayer position, you can try to extend the arms so that the top arm reaches towards the ceiling and the bottom arm to the floor. If you can't reach the floor with the bottom hand, then use a block for support. This is also a variation that you can practise with the back knee down on the floor.

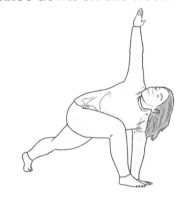

WHAT DOES IT DO?

Revolved side angle stretches and strengthens the legs and hips. It also stretches the chest and shoulders.

Like other twisting postures, revolved side angle stretches and strengthens the abdominal muscles and improves the mobility of the spine. It stimulates the abdominal organs and digestive system.

WHEN YOU SHOULDN'T DO IT

Avoid or modify this posture if you have a leg, hip, knee or shoulder injury. This posture is also usually not recommended if you have either high or low blood pressure.

STANDING WIDE LEG FORWARD FOLD

Prasarita padottanasana

Widening the stance in a forward fold changes how the hip joint moves. For some this can make the forward fold more accessible, for others it can be just as hard. The key is to approach the posture with patience and awareness. If you are more flexible, your focus will need to be on stability, if you feel more restricted in your range of motion look for the space that the breath can provide.

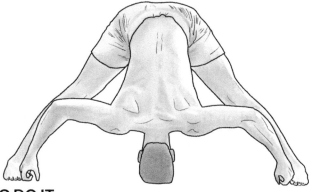

HOW TO DO IT

▷ Start in Mountain pose.

▷ Step your legs wide apart about 4 or 4 and a half feet.

▷ Make sure that your toes are pointing forward, rather than out to the sides.

▷ Put your hands on your hips.

▷ As you inhale, open your chest and lengthen the spine.

▷ As you exhale, fold forward at the hips, trying to maintain the length in the spine.

▷ Place your fingertips or hands on the floor underneath the shoulders.

▷ As you inhale, engage the core and lengthen the spine.

▷ As you exhale, try and bring the crown of the head

towards the floor.

▷ Catch hold of your big toes with the first two fingers of each hand, bend the elbows and draw the shoulder blades away from the ears.

▷ Hold the posture for 30 seconds or several long slow breaths.

▷ Come out of the posture the same way that you went into it.

If you find it hard enough just to get your hands on the floor, stay there – there's no need to try and grab the big toes and force the stretch. If you can't get your hands on the floor at all, or your back feels uncomfortable going into the posture, you can put your hands on blocks directly underneath your shoulders.

If you have very tight hamstrings and you find that your back rounds very quickly, you can bend your knees slightly to help you fold more from the hip joints.

Pay attention to where you feel your bodyweight in your feet - try and spread the weight evenly over the whole foot. That often means bringing it forward out of your heels.

WHAT DOES IT DO?

Standing wide leg forward fold stretches the legs and back, in particular the hamstrings and inner thighs. It improves the flexibility of the hips.

The posture also acts as a kind of mild inversion because it brings your heart above your head, which can bring you some of the benefits that inversions confer and can have an incredibly calming effect.

WHEN YOU SHOULDN'T DO IT

If you have lower back pain or a spinal injury, approach the posture with extreme caution. That can mean using blocks under your hands, or even avoiding it completely Likewise, if you have a leg, knee or hip injury you might need to modify or avoid the posture completely.

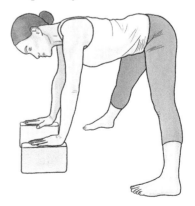

97

INTENSE SIDE STRETCH POSE

Parsvottanasana

This pose is often called Pyramid pose because of the shape of the legs. The Sanskrit translates as Intense side stretch pose which isn't nearly as catchy but explains a little bit about what you're trying to do in the posture. The aim is to lengthen and stretch the spine, although to begin with, you'll feel the most intense sensation in the hamstrings and hips.

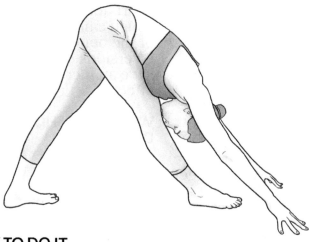

HOW TO DO IT

▷ Start in Mountain pose.

▷ Put your hands on your hips and step your left foot back about 3 to 3 and half feet.

▷ Turn your left foot out to a 45-degree angle so you can keep your back heel on the floor. Try to keep the heels in one line.

▷ Try and keep both hips facing forward - notice that with your back leg stepped back, the pelvis might have changed position.

▷ Inhale and lengthen the spine, almost like you're going to do a backbend.

▷ As you exhale, fold forward from the waist, trying to keep the spine from rounding while keeping the legs straight.

- ▷ Place your hands on the floor either side of your right foot.

- ▷ Stretch your spine forwards over your front leg.

- ▷ Hold the posture for 30 seconds or several long slow breaths.

- ▷ Repeat on the other side.

NOTES & ALTERNATIVES

If you can't reach the floor with your hands without rounding the spine, then use blocks. Alternatively you can put your hands on your front shin, although this will feel less stable.

If it feels that the posture is straining the knee of the front leg, then keep a tiny bend in it. That will help to engage the hamstring of the front leg which will help to feel like the knee is not taking so much pressure.

As with all these standing postures with the feet apart, if you find the position of the hips very challenging and uncomfortable, practise it with the feet set wider side to side (see 'A short note on feet').

TO CHALLENGE YOURSELF

Eventually as your hamstrings get more flexible, you can bring your hands further forward of your front foot and bring your chin towards your shin, so that your whole spine is stretching over your front leg. Don't be in a hurry to do this, as often instead of the spine stretching forward, it will round as you try to bring the body down.

A more challenging variation is to start at the top with the hands in reverse prayer position behind your back (see next page). This requires considerable shoulder flexibility, but also can be modified (see 'Shoulder movements in Diamond pose' above). Practise the posture the same way, keeping your hands behind your back. This variation will put more load onto the front leg hamstring, so will strengthen it at the same time as lengthening the muscle.

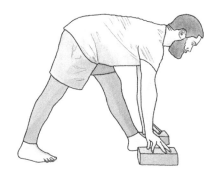

INTENSE SIDE STRETCH POSE
CONTINUED

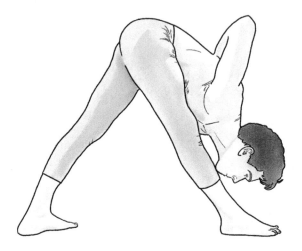

WHAT DOES IT DO?

Intense side stretch pose stretches and strengthens the legs and hips, in particular the hamstring of the front leg. By stretching the spine forward, you stretch the whole back of the body from the heel of the front foot to the neck as one connected chain, which is what makes the posture so effective.

It stimulates the abdominal organs and digestive system.

It also improves balance and stability.

WHEN YOU SHOULDN'T DO IT

If you have a back injury, avoid or modify the posture. Likewise, if you have a leg or hip injury.

This posture is also usually not recommended if you have either high or low blood pressure.

CHAPTER 7
POSTURES FOR GETTING STRONGER

Almost all the yoga postures covered so far in this book will build strength in one way or another, often in unexpected ways.

There are some postures that will work particularly well to develop strength: arm balances, preparation for inversions and core strengtheners.

CROW POSE

Kakasana

Crow pose is often the first arm balance that anyone learns. It involves carrying the whole weight of the body on the arms, and even if you only manage it for a moment, it's a great accomplishment!

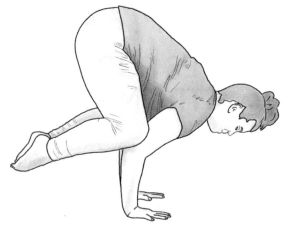

HOW TO DO IT

▷ Stand with the feet open at about shoulder-width distance.

▷ Bend your knees to lower yourself down into a squat.

▷ When you're low enough down to reach the floor, put your hands on the mat, shoulder width apart.

▷ Open the fingers so they're not squashed together.

▷ Come onto your tiptoes to raise the hips and put your knees on the back of the arms above the elbows, as high as possible.

▷ Bend the elbows and lean forward, lifting your hips up higher.

▷ Focus on a single point on the floor in front of you.

▷ Keep shifting your bodyweight forward until you can lift your feet off the ground.

- ▷ Keep trying to pull your knees up towards your armpits, and your heels towards your hips.

- ▷ Hold the posture for several long slow breaths or up to 30 seconds.

NOTES & ALTERNATIVES

To begin with you might not be able to lift your feet off the floor. If that's the case, don't worry and don't give up! Try and shift your bodyweight forward so that you feel the weight in your hands and hold that position for several breaths. Continue to practise it this way, holding for longer periods of time, so that you develop the strength to be able to lift yourself up. This will take some perseverance and determination.

One way of approaching the posture if you find it difficult is to start up higher, so there's less distance to travel to get onto your hands. You can start with your feet on one or two yoga blocks - the higher up you start, the easier the posture will be.

TO CHALLENGE YOURSELF

Try and practise the posture with straight arms. This is considerably more challenging than with bent arms, so approach it slowly and make sure that your wrists are well warmed up before you try it.

Alternatively, you could try to lift one of your legs up in the air, so that you practise a One-leg crow pose. These are both very challenging variations.

WHAT DOES IT DO?

Crow pose strengthens the core (particularly the hip flexors and abdominal muscles), arms and shoulders and stretches the upper back. It helps to develop balance and build confidence.

WHEN YOU SHOULDN'T DO IT

Avoid Crow pose if you have a wrist injury or are suffering from carpal tunnel syndrome, and practise with caution if you have an arm or shoulder injury.

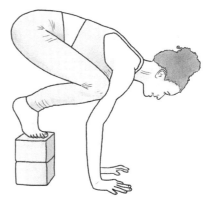

SIDE PLANK

Vasisthasana

As well as strengthening your arms and shoulders, Side plank will activate and engage your core. It's a great posture to practise to warm yourself up for a strength training workout, or to include as part of a powerful yoga sequence.

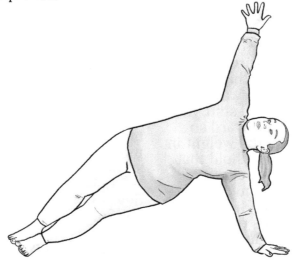

HOW TO DO IT

▷ Start in Downward dog.

▷ Press through the right hand and push up through the shoulder.

▷ Roll onto the outside edge of your right foot and stack your left foot on top of your right foot.

▷ Turn your body to face the left side of the mat and bring your left hand onto your left hip.

▷ Keep pressing strongly through the right hand on the mat. The right hand should be slightly in front of the shoulder, rather than directly underneath.

▷ Simultaneously push the hips up towards the ceiling and press the outer edge of the right foot against the floor.

▷ Stretch your left arm up towards the ceiling and look

at your left hand.

▷ Hold the posture for 30 seconds or several long slow breaths.

▷ Repeat on the other side.

NOTES & ALTERNATIVES

Just like with Plank pose, if your wrists hurt or you're suffering from carpal tunnel syndrome, you can practise this on your forearms. Make sure that you start with the forearm perpendicular to the body as this will provide the greatest support.

To begin with, you might feel that you don't have the strength to hold the posture for very long, or even at all. If that's the case, then you can bend the bottom knee and use it for support on the mat. This will also help to take the pressure off the supporting wrist.

If the balance is particularly challenging, then you don't need to stack the feet and can have them side by side to provide more support.

If your neck feels uncomfortable, then keep it neutral rather than looking at the top hand.

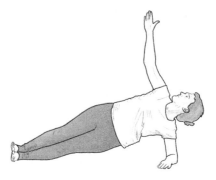

TO CHALLENGE YOURSELF:

Once you get the hang of the balance and develop the strength in the arms and shoulders to hold yourself up there easily, try and lift the top leg off the bottom leg. The higher you lift the leg, the harder it will be.

WHAT DOES IT DO?

Side plank strengthens the wrists, arms and shoulders. It stretches one side and strengthens the other side of the body, working the core muscles, particularly the obliques. Strengthening the obliques can be especially beneficial for your spine.

WHEN YOU SHOULDN'T DO IT

Avoid the posture if you have a serious wrist, elbow or shoulder injury.

FOREARM DOWNWARD DOG

Makarasana

This is a more challenging version of Downward dog that simultaneously strengthens and opens the shoulders. It's a great foundation for future work on inversions.

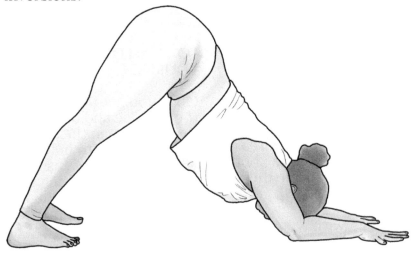

HOW TO DO IT

▷ Start on all fours, with hips over knees and hands under shoulders.

▷ Bring your forearms onto the floor so that the elbows are directly underneath the shoulders. Press the forearms and hands firmly into the mat.

▷ Curl your toes underneath so you can press through the balls of your feet and start to lift the hips up.

▷ Keep the knees bent to start with and try to lengthen the lower spine by untucking the pelvis.

▷ Gradually straighten the legs, engaging the core continuously.

▷ Try to resist the tendency of the shoulders to travel forwards in space by pressing through the forearms and drawing the shoulder blades down the back.

▷ Look at a point in between your arms on the mat.

▷ Hold the posture for 30 seconds or several long slow breaths.

NOTES & ALTERNATIVES

It doesn't matter whether you can get the legs straight or not - don't force it if your hamstrings feel tight. Similarly, don't worry if your heels don't reach the floor, even if they normally do in Downward dog. You'll get all the benefits of the posture through your shoulders even with the knees bent and the heels up.

If the neck feels uncomfortable, you can keep it more neutral and look back towards your feet, but make sure that your head isn't pushing against the floor.

TO CHALLENGE YOURSELF

Lift one leg off the floor into a 3-leg Forearm downward dog.

WHAT DOES IT DO?

Forearm downward dog stretches and strengthens the shoulders. It also stretches the legs, in particular the calves and hamstrings.

Like Downward dog, this posture is a mild inversion because it brings your heart above your head and gives some of the benefits to the nervous system and cardiovascular system that inversions provide.

WHEN YOU SHOULDN'T DO IT

If you have a shoulder, neck or arm injury avoid this posture. If your hamstrings feel tight, make sure that you keep the legs bent to start with, and pay attention to how your back feels when you practise it. You shouldn't feel stress or tension in the lower spine.

BOAT POSE

Navasana

Boat pose strengthens the core like no other posture, because it specifically focuses on your hip flexors, and although it can be challenging, there's a variation that should work for almost anyone!

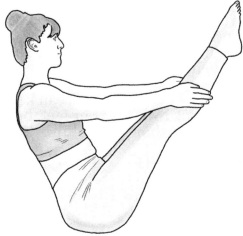

HOW TO DO IT:

▷ Start sitting on your mat with the knees bent and the feet together.

▷ Lean the upper body back and engage the abdominals to lengthen the spine so that it doesn't arch or round.

▷ Support the back of your thighs with your hands and lift the feet off the floor.

▷ Extend the arms alongside the legs so they're parallel to the floor.

▷ Gradually extend the legs so that they are roughly a 45-degree angle to the floor.

▷ Keep the core engaged while trying to maintain the length in the spine, so that the spine doesn't round.

▷ Hold the posture for 30 seconds or several long slow breaths.

▷ Repeat on the other side.

NOTES & ALTERNATIVES

The great thing about Boat pose is that you can stop at any point in the progression of the posture depending on how challenging you're finding it. To begin with you can try and balance while holding the thighs with the knees bent, as you get used to the position of the body and the legs.

Once you can balance easily, let go of the thighs, and keep the knees bent and the arms alongside your knees. The journey from bent knees to straight legs can also be challenging, and you can start by extending one leg at a time - hold each leg for half the time you would for the whole posture. That way you can progressively build the strength to hold the full posture.

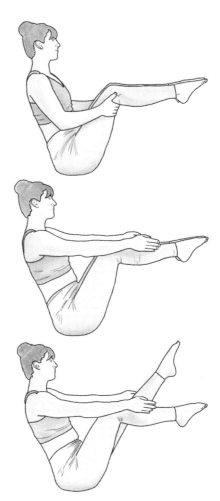

TO CHALLENGE YOURSELF

Try the posture lifting the arms overhead.

WHAT DOES IT DO?

Boat pose works the core in that it particularly strengthens the abdominals, the hip flexors and the lower spine.

It's a great posture for increasing focus and improving coordination and balance.

WHEN YOU SHOULDN'T DO IT

If you have serious hip or lower back injuries, avoid or modify the posture.

Boat pose is often not recommended for people who have significantly low blood pressure or heart problems.

CHAPTER 8
POSTURES TO INCREASE YOUR FOCUS

All yoga postures require concentration and focus in one way or another. But balancing on one leg will quickly make you concentrate because if you don't, you'll fall over.

Balance is also something that deteriorates over time, and it starts quite early on in life. From the age of about 25, balance steadily gets worse, unless you make efforts to maintain or improve it. Trying to balance by challenging your stability - even if you feel like you're not having much success - is the key. It sends the right stimulus to the nervous system to better process all the information it needs to keep you balanced.

TREE POSE

Vrksasana

Tree pose is a classic one leg balance which will help you to feel centred and grounded.

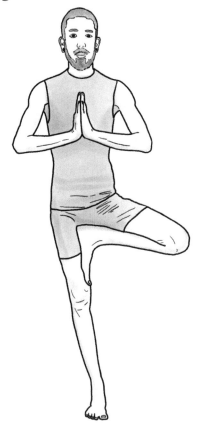

HOW TO DO IT

▷ Start in Mountain pose.

▷ Shift your weight to your left foot and bend your right knee.

▷ Bring your right knee out to the right, and the sole of your right foot up onto your inner thigh - you can use your hand to do this.

▷ Bring your hands in front of your chest in a prayer position.

▷ Focus your attention on a single point in front of you.

▷ Hold the posture for up to a minute or several long slow breaths.

▷ Repeat on the other side.

Don't worry about how high the foot of the bent knee goes up the inner thigh of the standing leg. Eventually it might reach up to your hips, but to begin with, especially if the knee feels uncomfortable, keep the foot lower down. If the balance is very challenging, to begin with you can even put the foot of the bent leg on the floor as a support like a kickstand.

If your standing leg knee feels sensitive, make sure you're not putting too much pressure from your lifted foot against it. You can also have a micro bend in it if that feels more comfortable. At the same time, try and contract the quadriceps, the big muscle group on the front of the thigh. That means that the

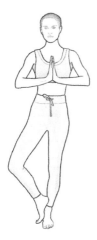

arms are over your head, you can bring the hands into a prayer position and change your gaze to look at your thumbs to really challenge your balance.

knee might not look bent from the outside, but you're not pushing the joint back as far as possible.

TO CHALLENGE YOURSELF

Try to bring your two knees in one line from the side. That usually means bringing your bent knee back in space so that there is an increase in hip abduction and external rotation in the same hip. The challenge is to make sure that the position of the pelvis doesn't change while you do this. In other words, try and keep the pelvis squared to the front of your mat.

Once you are more comfortable with the balance, you can change the position of the arms and bring them over your head, or even into reverse prayer position. If your

WHAT DOES IT DO?

Like all one leg balancing postures, Tree pose strengthens the standing leg and improves balance. Tree pose also engages the core muscles which are needed for stability in the posture. It increases body awareness and can have a calming effect on the mind.

It can also improve the flexibility of the hip, as the lifted leg is externally rotated at the hip joint, stretching the inner thigh.

WHEN YOU SHOULDN'T DO IT

If you are suffering from vertigo or have some severe balance issues, use a wall or a similar appropriate support.

If you have any kind of knee injury or sensitivity, start with the foot of the bent leg much lower down the standing leg, so that the knee isn't so fully flexed.

WARRIOR 3

Virabhadrasana 3

Like the other warrior poses, Warrior 3 is a powerful posture that builds strength and confidence. When you can, try and approach the posture with a sense of humour as it can be no laughing matter on some days!

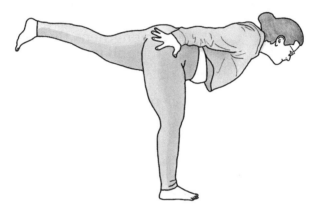

HOW TO DO IT

▷ Start in Mountain pose.

▷ Put your hands on your hips and shift your weight to your right foot.

▷ Hinge forward at your hips, bringing your torso down at the same time as lifting your left leg up.

▷ Bring your arms alongside your torso, angled slightly away from your body and draw your shoulder blades down your back.

▷ Try to bring your body down and the lifted leg up so that everything is parallel to the floor.

▷ Extend your back leg fully, flexing the foot and contracting the quadriceps.

▷ Try to keep both hips parallel to the floor, so that the toes of your back foot point down towards the ground.

▷ Focus on a single point on the floor in front of you.

▷ Hold the posture for 30 seconds or several long slow breaths. Repeat on the other side.

Bringing your body down parallel to the floor can be very challenging to begin with, and you should approach it slowly. Just go down as far as you can without rounding the spine - even if that's not very far to start with. Try and make sure that the movement is a hinge from the hips, rather than a rounding of the spine.

If you feel you can perform the movement but find you don't have the strength to hold yourself there for very long, then use some support - you can put your hands on a chair, or use blocks, so that you can build up your endurance. You can gradually reduce the support you need and try to hold the posture for longer without it.

Be aware of how the knee of your standing leg feels in the posture. Keep the quadriceps, the muscles on the front of the leg, contracted. However, if your knee feels sensitive, keep a slight bend in the standing leg.

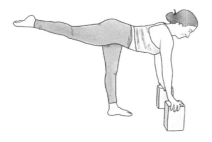

TO CHALLENGE YOURSELF

Try the posture with your arms over your head, either with the palms together or the hands at shoulder width.

WHAT DOES IT DO?

Warrior 3 strengthens the whole body, in particular the legs, hips and the ankles. As the hamstrings and glutes of the standing leg are being stretched under the load of your upper body, they get stronger in lengthened position. The glutes of the back leg are being used to lift the leg up and keep it there, so they get strengthened too.

Warrior 3 improves balance and can have a positive effect on posture. It can give you a boost of energy and alertness as it requires all your effort and attention to keep yourself in it.

WHEN YOU SHOULDN'T DO IT

This posture usually isn't recommended for people with very high blood pressure. If you have any knee, leg or hip injuries, approach the posture cautiously, using as much support as necessary.

HALF-MOON POSE

Ardha chandrasana

Half-moon pose is a bit like Triangle pose, only it's practised on one leg. The hip position is similar which means Triangle pose is often used in a sequence as the posture just before Half moon. Of course, there are lots of different ways to get into the posture, so the instructions below are from Mountain pose.

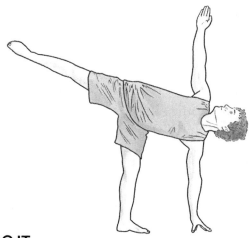

HOW TO DO IT

▷ Start in Mountain pose.

▷ Put your hands on your hips and shift your weight to your right foot.

▷ Hinge forward at your hips, bringing your torso down at the same time as lifting your left leg up, just like you would when practising Warrior 3.

▷ Bring your right hand down directly underneath your right shoulder and place your fingertips on the floor.

▷ Keeping your left hand on your left hip, rotate your left hip up towards the ceiling so that your body starts to turn out to the left.

▷ Extend your back leg and flex your back foot.

▷ Lift your left arm up and stretch it up towards the ceiling.

▷ Turn your head and look towards your left hand.

▷ Hold the posture for 30 seconds or several long slow breaths. Repeat on the other side.

NOTES & ALTERNATIVES

If your shoulder or neck feels uncomfortable, or the balance is challenging, you can keep your top hand on your hip and keep your focus on the floor, rather than turning your head.

If you can't reach the floor with your bottom hand, you have two options. The first is to bend the standing knee as much as you need to reach the floor, and work on the posture with the knee bent. This will mean you feel much less stable. The second is to use a block. Place it on the floor underneath your hand for support. As your flexibility and balance improves, you can lower the block.

Bear in mind when you practise the pose that it's not an arm balance. In other words, make sure that you're only using the hand or the fingertips for support and that most of your bodyweight is being carried by the standing leg.

Also be aware of how the knee of your standing leg feels in the posture. Keep the quadriceps (the muscles on the front of the leg) contracted. However, if your knee feels sensitive, keep a slight bend in the standing leg.

WHAT DOES IT DO?

Half-moon pose stretches and strengthens the legs and the hips, particularly stretching the hamstrings and strengthening the glutes of the standing leg.

It improves balance and coordination, while also activating and strengthening your core.

WHEN YOU SHOULDN'T DO IT

If you have any knee, leg or hip injuries, approach the posture cautiously, using as much support as necessary. This posture usually isn't recommended for people with low blood pressure.

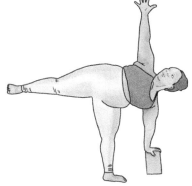

EXTENDED HAND TO BIG TOE

Uttitha hasta padangusthasana

Extended hand to big toe is quite a mouthful of a name. It's a multipart posture which takes balancing on one leg and hip mobility to the next level.

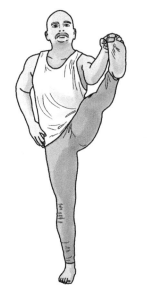

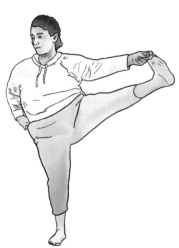

HOW TO DO IT

▷ Start in Mountain pose.

▷ Put your hands on your hips and shift your weight to your left foot.

▷ Bend your right knee and lift your leg to bring your thigh up as high as possible.

▷ Reach your right hand down and grip your right big toe with the first toe fingers of your right hand.

▷ Keep the spine straight and extend the right leg out in front of you.

▷ Find your balance and focus your attention on a single point in front of you.

▷ Bring your right leg out to the right. Try to keep the hips in one line facing the front of your mat.

▷ Look over your left shoulder.

▷ Hold the posture for 30 seconds or several long slow breaths.

▷ Bring the right leg back

to the centre, bend the knee and release the foot.

▷ Repeat on the other side.

NOTES & ALTERNATIVES

This posture can be especially challenging if you have very tight hamstrings, so you can start to practise it with the knee bent and hold onto the knee rather than the big toe. It's a great option if you really struggle to reach the big toe or extend the spine back straight once you've got a hold of it.

If you try to extend the leg of the foot that you're holding out in front of you and the spine rounds as you do so, or if you can't fully extend the leg, keep the leg bent. You can keep it bent as you abduct the hip and bring the leg out to the side. Alternatively, you can use a strap (if you don't have a strap, use a tea towel or a belt). Wrap it around the foot and hold onto it with your hand so that you can fully extend the knee while keeping the spine straight.

As with the other one leg balancing poses, be aware of how the knee of your standing leg feels in the posture. Keep the quadriceps (the muscles on the front of the leg) contracted. However, if your knee feels sensitive, keep a slight bend in the standing leg.

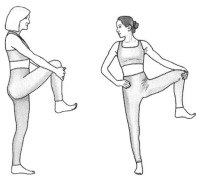

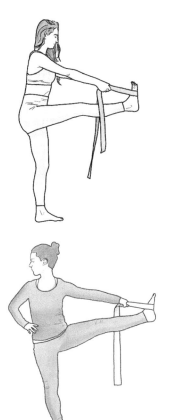

119

EXTENDED HAND TO BIG TOE
CONTINUED

If your neck feels uncomfortable, or you find the balance especially challenging, then don't turn your head.

TO CHALLENGE YOURSELF

Once you have done both parts of the posture, try holding the leg out in front of you without using your hand to keep it up. Don't worry if the leg drops a little (or a lot) from where you were holding it with your hand. Try to maintain the same position of your hips and spine when you let go of the foot. In other words, don't lean your upper body back to get the leg higher. If you find it really challenging, you can start with the knee bent and gradually straighten it as you get stronger. You can keep your hands on your hips or bring your arms up over your head.

WHAT DOES IT DO?

Extended hand to big toe pose stretches and strengthens the legs and hips. It particularly stretches the hamstrings and inner thighs while activating the hip stabilisers, & strengthens the standing leg.

Both parts of the posture challenge stability and therefore improve balance and proprioception. If you let go of the foot and try to hold the leg up its own, then you increase the strengthening effect on the hip flexor and quadriceps of the lifted leg.

WHEN YOU SHOULDN'T DO IT

If you're having serious balance issues, you can use the support of a chair or a wall.

Be careful with any ankle, knee or hip injury, and be extremely cautious with injuries to the lower back.

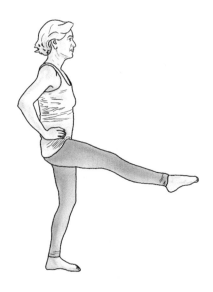

CHAPTER 9
POSTURES THAT MAKE YOU FEEL YOUNGER

The truth is that practising any of the postures detailed in this book will make you feel younger. However, there is one group of postures which will - if practised regularly - make you feel rejuvenated and energised in a unique way.

Backbends get the spine moving in a direction that they don't often move in, and movement is what keeps your body healthy. Keeping your spine healthy is the key to feeling young!

In an earlier chapter, we looked at two key back bending postures, Cobra pose and Upward facing dog, but there are many more which can be incorporated into a practice.

LOCUST POSE

Salabhasana

Locust pose fundamentally strengthens the back in a simple way. There are lots of different variations of the posture but most of them follow the same pattern: you lift your body up off the floor into an arched position using your back muscles. But just because it's simple doesn't mean it's easy! Practise this posture regularly and you'll feel the difference in your whole body.

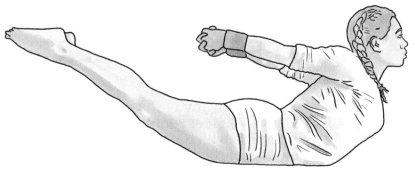

HOW TO DO IT

▷ Lie on your front with your legs about hip width apart.

▷ Bring your hand behind your back and interlace the fingers.

▷ As you exhale, lift your head, chest and legs off the floor. Try and lift your arms up off your hips as well and squeeze the shoulder blades together.

▷ You can keep the neck neutral or gently arch it back in line with the rest of the spine.

▷ Contract the glutes, and also contract the thigh muscles, to keep the legs extended.

▷ Hold the posture for 30 seconds or several long slow breaths.

NOTES & ALTERNATIVES

If you can't reach your hands together behind your back, you can put something in between them. If you have a yoga strap use that, but anything will work - you can use a tea towel or t-shirt. If bringing your arms behind your back is really uncomfortable, you can practise the posture with the arms by your sides.

If your neck feels uncomfortable, don't lift your head up. Instead look at the floor while you're in the posture.

TO CHALLENGE YOURSELF

Try bringing the arms straight out in front of you so that you look a bit like superman. If you want to make it really hard, hold a yoga block between your hands when they're stretched out in front of you.

WHAT DOES IT DO?

Locust pose strengthens the back muscles, it particularly strengthens the deep muscles which extend the spine. It also activates the muscles of the legs and hips.

With the hands behind the back, it stretches the chest, shoulders. It can stimulate the abdominal organs as it stretches the abdomen.

WHEN YOU SHOULDN'T DO IT

If you have a back injury that means you can't extend the spine, avoid the posture until the injury has healed.

If you have a headache avoid backward bending postures.

BOW POSE

Dhanurasana

As BKS Iyengar famously said about yoga, "Body is the bow. Asana is the arrow. Soul is the target." And you can see where Bow pose gets its name from, here the body literally is a bow. The posture powerfully stretches the front of the body, using the strength of your own legs.

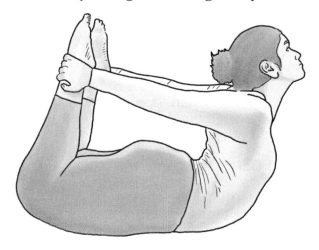

HOW TO DO IT

▷ Lie on your front with your legs about hip width apart and your arms by your sides.

▷ Bend your knees and bring your heels as close to your hips as possible.

▷ Reach your arms back behind you and grab your feet, holding them from the outside.

▷ Start to lift the heels away from your hips by extending the legs, strongly pressing the feet into the hands.

▷ Arch the spine back and up - the body will be pulled up by extending the legs.

▷ You can keep the neck neutral or gently arch it back in line with the rest of the spine.

▷ Hold the posture for 30 seconds or several long slow breaths.

To begin with, if you have a lot of difficulty in grabbing the feet because the quadriceps or shoulders are tight, you can try the posture on one side at a time. Sometimes this can give you more space to reach the foot. Keep the forearm of the other arm on the floor as a support to lift the chest up.

You can either grab the ankles or the tops of the feet. Try both grips and notice if you feel a difference in the shoulders or the ease of the backbend between the two.

WHAT DOES IT DO?

Bow pose stretches the whole front of the body, especially the hip flexors and shoulders. It also strongly activates the spinal muscles. It can stimulate the abdominal organs.

WHEN YOU SHOULDN'T DO IT

If you have a back injury that means you can't extend the spine, avoid the posture until the injury has healed. Be careful with any injuries of the shoulders and knees and approach the posture slowly.

"I am not what happened to me, I am what I choose to become."

CARL JUNG

CAMEL POSE

Ustrasana

Whereas in bow pose and locust you are using the body
as a weight to lift against the force of gravity, Camel
pose works in the other direction. Gravity is on your
side, which means the posture not only improves the
flexibility of the spine but also stretches and
strengthens the front of the body.

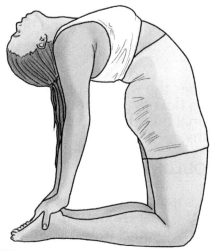

HOW TO DO IT

▷ Start kneeling on the floor with your knees and feet
hip distance apart.

▷ Keep the tops of the feet flat on the floor and press
them down evenly.

▷ Put your hands on your lower back, just above your
hips, with the fingers pointing down.

▷ Lengthen the tailbone down to keep the pelvis in a
neutral position.

▷ As you inhale, lift the chest up, start to backward
bend the spine and extend the hips. Keep the hips
stacked above the knees.

▷ Bring your hands from your back to your heels, one
at a time for support.

▷ Keep pushing the chest up and gently bring your head back.

▷ Hold the posture for 30 seconds or several long slow breaths.

Come out of the posture by bringing your hands back to your lower back one at a time before you straighten up the spine.

If you can't reach the feet with your hands, then curl your toes underneath, so that the heels are a little higher. This might enable you to reach them - even if you can only get your fingertips on them for support. If you can't reach your feet at all, or you find the movement too intense, keep your hands on your lower back for support.

If your neck feels sensitive, then you don't need to drop the head all the way back. A good way to practise the posture is to keep your neck in line with the rest of your spine. That way you can use your head as a weight to strengthen the muscles of your neck as you start to arch your spine back.

You can also put padding underneath your knees if they feel uncomfortable from the pressure as you go back into the posture.

WHAT DOES IT DO?

Camel pose stretches the whole front of your body. At the same time, it also works to strengthen the muscles of the front of the body - the hip flexors and abdominals - to support the backbend. It improves spinal mobility and activates the spinal muscles.

Stretching the shoulders and chest can help to improve posture. Stretching the front of the body stimulates the abdominal organs.

WHEN YOU SHOULDN'T DO IT

If you have serious neck or back injuries, approach the posture very cautiously. To begin with you can just keep your hands on your lower back and move the spine minimally.

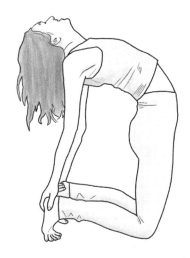

SPHINX POSE

Salamba bhujangasana

Sphinx pose is a great posture to get started with backbends as you have a lot of support from the arms and the floor. It's a less intense version of Cobra pose, allowing your body to understand the mechanics of what you're doing before going deeper.

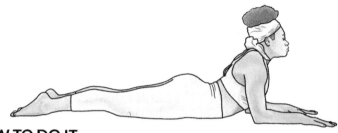

HOW TO DO IT

▷ Lie on your front with your legs about hip width apart.

▷ Bring your elbows to the floor underneath your shoulders and the forearms parallel to each other.

▷ Lengthen the tailbone down, so that you're not overly arching the lower spine.

▷ Draw your chest up and forward, whilst pulling the shoulder blades down your back.

▷ Hold the posture for 30 seconds or several long slow breaths.

WHAT DOES IT DO?

Sphinx pose has all the same kind of benefits as Cobra pose, just to a lesser degree. It strengthens and mobilises the spine and it stretches the chest, shoulders and abdomen. It can stimulate the abdominal organs.

WHEN YOU SHOULDN'T DO IT

If you have a back injury that means you can't extend the spine, avoid the posture until the injury has healed. If you have a headache avoid backward bending postures.

CHAPTER 10
POSTURES THAT KEEP YOU FEELING FLEXIBLE

Pretty much all yoga postures will help with your flexibility in one way or another. However, that doesn't mean you'll always feel at your most flexible. Nowhere does this feel more apparent than when you are sitting on the floor. Because we spend so much time sitting in chairs, sitting on the floor can feel very difficult. This collection of seated postures will help make time on the floor more comfortable.

STAFF POSE

Dandasana

Staff pose looks deceptively easy, but it can be very challenging, depending on the flexibility of your hips and hamstrings. It's a great preparation for the postures which follow.

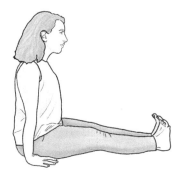

HOW TO DO IT

▷ Sit on the floor with your legs together and extended out in front of you.

▷ Flex your feet, so the toes start to point back towards your face.

▷ Keep your arms by your sides, palms facing down on the floor, fingers pointing towards the feet.

▷ Gently press the palms against the floor to lengthen the spine up towards the ceiling.

▷ Hold the posture for up to a minute or several long slow breaths.

If your hips or hamstrings are tight, and you feel that your torso is leaning backwards, then sit on something to raise the hips up. Use a folded blanket or a yoga block to bring your spine more perpendicular to the floor.

WHAT DOES IT DO?

Staff pose gently stretches the back of the legs, and the chest and shoulders. It activates the thigh muscles when you extend the legs and can help to strengthen some of the postural muscles of your back. It helps to realign the relationship between your hips, hamstrings and spine in an active seated position.

WHEN YOU SHOULDN'T DO IT

If you have a lower back injury, avoid the posture until the injury has healed. If you have a wrist injury, you can use your fingertips or put your hands in another position that doesn't exacerbate the injury.

SEATED FORWARD FOLD

Paschimottanasana

The Seated forward fold is called *Paschimottanasana* in Sanskrit which translates as "intense stretch of the west." One suggested reasoning for this is that traditionally you would practise in the morning facing the sun in the east. This pose stretches the whole back of the body which would therefore be facing the west.

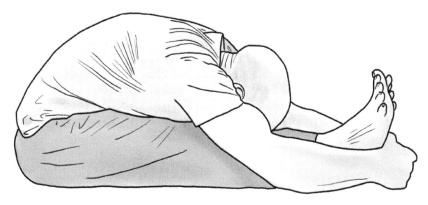

HOW TO DO IT

▷ Start in Staff pose.

▷ Inhale and lengthen the torso as much as possible.

▷ As you exhale, hinge forward from the hips.

▷ Try and keep the spine as straight as possible as you fold over the thighs.

▷ Take hold of the side of your feet with your hands.

▷ Look forward at your feet.

▷ As you inhale, try to lengthen the torso, and as you exhale fold over the legs, even if the movements are very small.

▷ Hold the posture for up to a minute or several long slow breaths.

SEATED FORWARD FOLD
CONTINUED

NOTES & ALTERNATIVES

To begin with, you might feel it is impossible to keep lengthening the torso as you fold over the legs. Instead, you might find that the spine just rounds, and you end up looking at your knees. If this happens, there are two options you could try.

First, you can bend the knees. That way you can more easily reach your feet. At the same time, with the knees bent, it is easier to keep the pelvis into a forward tilt. In other words, you'll be able to keep the spine straighter because it won't be being pulled back by the pelvis. You can then work on gradually straightening the legs, while maintaining the position of the hips and the stretch of the spine.

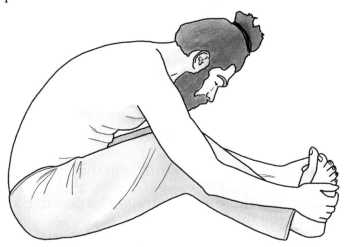

Second, you can use props. Just like with Staff pose, if you raise the hips up, it's much easier to change the position of the pelvis and stop it feeling like it is so tucked underneath. If you can't reach your feet, use something to help you. If you have a yoga strap you can use that. If you don't have one, anything that you can hook over your feet - like a hand towel - will work just as well.

Don't be in a hurry to go deep into the forward bend. If you find Staff pose challenging, then this pose will just

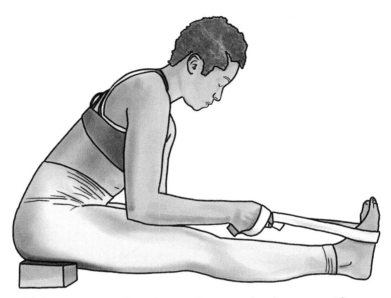

be a slight progression from there - don't worry if your torso is quite upright and you feel you need to use lots of props to make the movement more comfortable.

WHAT DOES IT DO?

Seated forward fold stretches the whole back of the body, in particular the calves, hamstrings and lower back. It also stretches the shoulders when they're in the overhead position, so that will depend on how low you can bring your body down. The posture also aims to lengthen and stretch the entire spine.

In general, forward bends can be very calming. Seated forward fold can also support a whole range of mental benefits, like helping to relieve stress, reduce anxiety and fatigue.

WHEN YOU SHOULDN'T DO IT

If you've got very tight hamstrings, make sure that you modify the posture appropriately. If you have any spinal injuries or lower back problems, approach the posture very cautiously or avoid it entirely until the injury has been resolved.

REVERSE PLANK

Purvottanasana

Reverse plank is the ideal counterpose to the Seated forward fold. After stretching the back of the body, you then contract it strongly to lift the body up off the floor. It's also a great counterpose for Low-level plank, for the opposite reason - it stretches the areas that Low-level plank works.

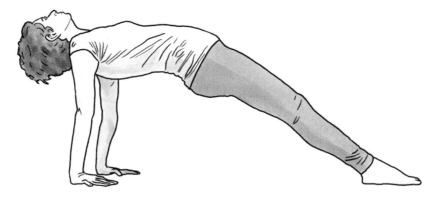

HOW TO DO IT

▷ Start in Staff pose.

▷ Put your hands on the floor about 6 inches behind your hips, with the fingers facing forward.

▷ Press firmly through your palms and lift your hips as high as possible.

▷ Roll the thighs in towards each other and draw in the abdomen.

▷ Try to straighten the legs and point your toes forward to bring them down towards the floor.

▷ Lift your chest up and gently arch your neck back.

▷ Hold the posture for 30 seconds or several long slow breaths.

NOTES & ALTERNATIVES

If your neck feels uncomfortable, then don't drop the neck back - always go slowly with any neck movements.

If you can't lift the body off the floor with straight legs, then keep the knees bent and have the heels under the knees. You can also start with the knees bent and try to extend the legs one at a time.

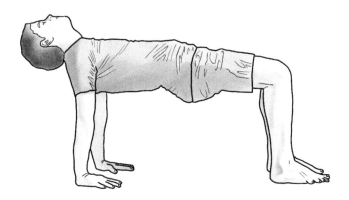

WHAT DOES IT DO?

It strengthens the arms and legs and activates the whole back of the body. It also stretches the chest and shoulders, and the tops of the ankles, when you try to bring the toes to the floor. It helps to build core strength and awareness.

WHEN YOU SHOULDN'T DO IT

Avoid this posture if you have a wrist injury, carpal tunnel syndrome or a shoulder injury.

"Thousands of candles can be lighted from a single candle, and the life of the candle will not be shortened. Happiness never decreases by being shared."

BUDDHA

HEAD TO KNEE POSE

Janu Sirsasana

Although this posture is called Head to knee, you don't actually have to bring your head to your knee. In fact, as you get more flexible, your aim is to bring the head onto the leg somewhere beyond the knee.

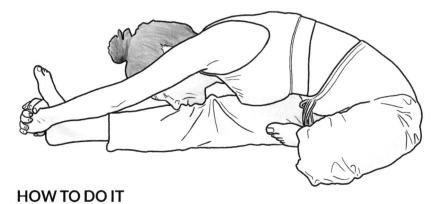

HOW TO DO IT

▷ Start in Staff pose.

▷ Bend your right knee and place the sole of your right foot on the inner thigh close to your groin.

▷ Turn your body slightly to the left so that your navel lines up with the middle of your left thigh.

▷ As you inhale, reach your arms up to lengthen your torso.

▷ As you exhale, fold over your left leg and catch hold of your left foot.

▷ Keep the neck in line with the rest of the spine and lengthen your spine over your left leg.

▷ Hold the posture for up to a minute or several long slow breaths.

If the knee of your folded leg doesn't reach the floor or feels uncomfortable, put something underneath to support it.

As with all forward bends, make sure that you're not rounding your spine. Try to make sure the movement feels more like a hinge at the hips. That might mean you need to stay much higher up, which is fine - there's no hurry to bring your head to your shin. Think first of trying to bring the stomach to touch the thigh before the head reaches the leg.

Just like the Seated forward fold, if you feel that your hips and hamstrings are quite tight and that sitting on the floor is difficult, raise the hips up by sitting on a folded blanket or a low yoga block. If you can't reach the feet then use a prop, like a yoga strap or a hand towel to wrap around the feet. That way you'll find it easier to keep lengthening the spine.

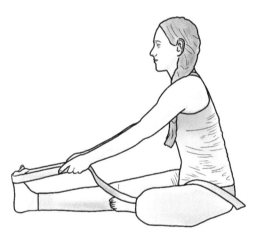

WHAT DOES IT DO?

Head to knee pose stretches the hamstrings, hips, spine. It stretches the shoulders when the arms are over the head. Like all the forward bends, Head to knee pose can be very calming. Practising it regularly can help to relieve stress, reduce anxiety and fatigue.

WHEN YOU SHOULDN'T DO IT

If you have a knee injury, be careful with the knee that you're bending. You do not have to fully flex the knee and can always support the knee as much as necessary.

As with all forward bending postures, if you have any spinal injuries or lower back problems, approach the posture very cautiously or avoid it until the injury has been resolved.

SEATED SPINAL TWIST

Ardha matsyendrasana

The direct translation of *Ardha matsyendrasana* is "Half lord of the fishes pose," which is a reference to one of the early figures in Hatha Yoga who, according to legend, was swallowed by a fish when he was a baby. He learnt the secrets of yoga which he practised in the fish's belly

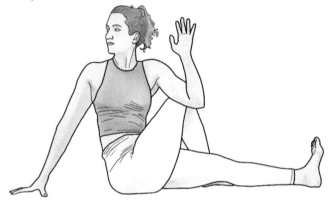

HOW TO DO IT

▷ Start in Staff pose.

▷ Bend the right knee and place the foot on the outside edge of the left knee, so that the right knee points up towards the ceiling.

▷ Keep both sitting bones grounded on the floor.

▷ Put your right hand on the floor behind your hips, with the fingers pointing to the back.

▷ As you inhale, lift your left arm and lengthen the spine. Use the arm behind your back to help keep the spine up straight.

▷ As you exhale, twist your torso to the right. Bend your left arm and bring your elbow on the outside edge of the right knee.

▷ Press the elbow against the side of the leg and press the side of the leg back against the elbow.

▷ Start to twist the torso more to the right, turn your

head and look over the right shoulder.

▷ As you inhale, lengthen the spine, pushing your hand against the floor, and as you exhale twist.

▷ Hold the posture for 30 seconds or several long slow breaths.

If you have trouble keeping the spine upright, raising the hips up can help - sit on a folded blanket or a low yoga block. If you feel restricted in the hips, you don't need to cross the foot onto the other side of the knee, keep it on the inside.

If you feel restricted in the twist, and you can't reach the elbow onto the other side of the top knee, then you can use your arm to hold onto the leg. Wrap your arm around the leg so that you can hug it into your torso. That will also help you to lengthen the spine which will assist with the twist.

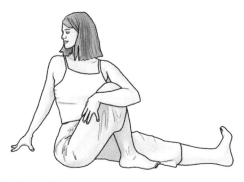

WHAT DOES IT DO?

Spinal twists improve the spine by keeping it mobile. Twists also stimulate the abdominal organs and digestive system.

The abdominal muscles - in particular the obliques - are the muscles which help rotate the spine, so this posture also activates and strengthens the obliques as they are helping to maintain the spine in an upright position.

WHEN YOU SHOULDN'T DO IT

If you have a back or spine injury, avoid the posture until the injury has been resolved.

CHAPTER 11
POSTURES FOR WINDING DOWN

Not all yoga can seem relaxing. If you've practised some of the other postures in this book, you'll quickly see how challenging they can be, and how much effort they involve. Depending on how fast you move, you can even build up some heat in the body and start sweating.

The overall effect, of course, is one of relaxation, and that's where this next set of postures comes in. They are a great way to finish a practice, or even postures just to practise in themselves. If you need to wind down and relax, holding them each for a minute or so each would have a great effect.

BRIDGE

Setu bandha sarvangasana

Bridge is a supine back bending posture. Supine means lying on your back. Most backbends strongly stimulate the nervous system. However, Bridge provides a lot of support, and it can have some of the same effects as an inversion. So, while it can be rejuvenating and invigorating, it can also be practised in a way that is restorative and relaxing.

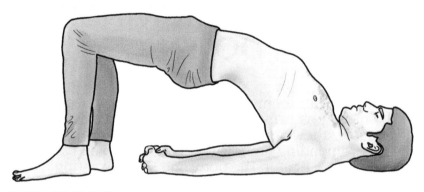

HOW TO DO IT

▷ Start lying on your back with your palms facing down.

▷ Bend your knees and put your feet flat on the floor, so that the heels are underneath the knees, and the feet are hip distance apart.

▷ Pushing through your hands and your feet, lift the hips up off the floor until the thighs are more or less parallel to the floor.

▷ Lengthen the tailbone down to keep the pelvis neutral.

▷ Keep the knees and feet the same distance apart throughout the posture.

▷ Bring your arms behind your back and interlace the fingers.

▷ Push through your arms against the floor and lift your chest up.

▷ Hold the posture for up to a minute or several long slow breaths.

NOTES & ALTERNATIVES

Notice where your body weight is centred through the feet during the posture. Make sure that it is not concentrated on one edge - particularly the outer edge - try to spread the pressure over the whole of the foot.

If you're having trouble keeping the hips up in the air, or you want to make the posture truly relaxing, then prop yourself up. Use a yoga block or bolster underneath your hips - or if you don't have one, a stack of cushions will work just as well.

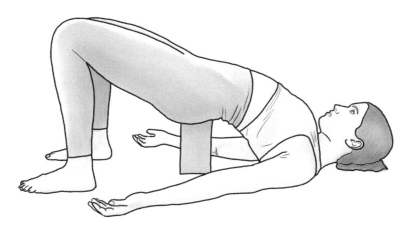

TO CHALLENGE YOURSELF

Try and lift one leg off the floor in the air while keeping the hips up off the floor.

WHAT DOES IT DO?

Bridge stretches the chest, shoulders, abdomen and hip flexors. It also stretches the back of the neck - the higher you lift the chest up, the greater the effect.

WHEN YOU SHOULDN'T DO IT

If you've got a neck or a spine injury, approach the posture with caution. Avoid it especially if the pressure on the neck feels too great.

143

WIND RELIEVING POSE

Pavanamuktasana

Wind relieving pose is one of the simplest postures, yet when you practise it regularly it can have a very powerful effect. It's one of the best examples of a common principle in yoga, that you don't have to do extreme things or crazy postures: doing something simple but consistently will see long term and profound change.

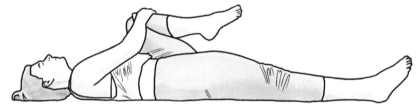

HOW TO DO IT

▷ Start lying on your back with both legs extended.

▷ Bend the right knee and bring it close to your chest.

▷ Grab your right shin, below the knee, and interlace your fingers.

▷ Pull the right knee down towards your right shoulder, avoiding the ribcage.

▷ Try and keep both shoulders on the floor evenly and your left leg extended and on the floor.

▷ Hold the posture for 30 seconds or several long slow breaths.

▷ Repeat on the left side.

▷ Once you've done both sides, bend both knees and bring them close to your chest.

▷ Wrap your arms around your legs and try to grab your elbows.

▷ Keep the head on the floor and bring the chin gently towards the chest to lengthen the back of your neck.

▷ Hold the posture for 30 seconds or several long slow breaths.

NOTES & ALTERNATIVES

If your knees hurt, you can't bend them fully or you can't reach your shins, you can grab the back of the leg around the hamstring instead.

When lifting both legs at the same time, you don't need to actively pull the legs in towards the chest. Just get the tightest grip that you can and think of slowly lengthening the spine on the floor. That means it doesn't matter if you can't reach your elbows. Just grab where you can and hold on!

If your head doesn't reach the floor or lifts when you try to grab both legs, you can put something underneath it for support, like a block or a book. Bear in mind that over time, you're likely to become more flexible from practice, which means you might not always need the support under your head.

WHAT DOES IT DO?

This posture primarily works on your digestive system, helping to regulate it by massaging the abdomen. The digestive system is increasingly being understood to be an important part of both your immune system and your mental wellbeing, so you can't underestimate the importance of keeping it healthy

WHEN YOU SHOULDN'T DO IT

If you have any spinal problems, approach this posture with caution or avoid it until the problems have become resolved. If you have a hernia, avoid this posture.

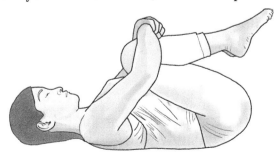

HAPPY BABY

Ananda balasana

This pose is a great way to relax and unwind and is the perfect recovery pose after a big cardio session or some heavy leg training.

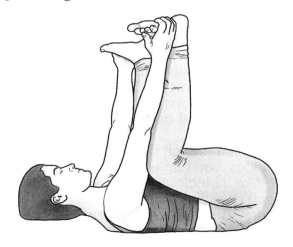

HOW TO DO IT

▷ Start lying on your back.

▷ As you exhale, bend your knees towards your chest and hold the outer edge of your feet with your hands.

▷ Open your knees out to the sides and pull your knees down towards your armpits.

▷ Flex your feet to bring the soles of your feet to face the ceiling, and the heels to stack over your knees, so that the shins are perpendicular to the floor.

▷ Hold the posture for up to a minute or several long slow breaths.

NOTES & ALTERNATIVES

If you can't reach the feet, you can use a prop, like a yoga belt or a tea towel hooked around them. If you don't have anything handy, you can just hold on to your shins or underneath your hamstrings instead.

Just like for Wind relieving pose, if your head doesn't rest comfortably on the floor, put something underneath it for support.

WHAT DOES IT DO?

Happy baby gently stretches the hips and inner thighs. It's a very relaxing posture which can help calm your mind.

WHEN YOU SHOULDN'T DO IT

If you have knee injuries which mean you can't flex the joint, wait until the injury is sufficiently recovered. If you have a back injury, approach the posture cautiously.

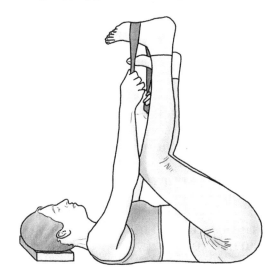

"The word 'yoga' means skill—skill to live your life, to manage your mind, to deal with your emotions, to be with people, to be in love, and not let that love turn into hatred."

SRI CHINMOY

RECLINED PIGEON

Supta kapotasana

This posture is sometimes called Thread the needle or even Dead pigeon, so you might have come across it before under a different name. It's a great way to work on hip flexibility.

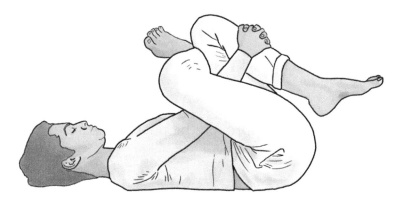

HOW TO DO IT

▷ Start lying on your back.

▷ Bend both knees and put your feet flat on the floor.

▷ Bring the ankle of your right leg onto the left thigh, just below your knee.

▷ Flex your right foot, and make sure the sole of the foot isn't turned towards you.

▷ Thread your right arm through the gap between your two legs and bring your left arm around the left side of your left leg.

▷ Interlace the fingers on the shin of your left leg.

▷ Gently pull your left knee towards your left shoulder.

▷ Hold the posture for up to a minute or several long slow breaths.

▷ Repeat on the other side.

NOTES & ALTERNATIVES

If you can't reach your shin, or if the only way you can reach is by lifting your upper body up off the floor, you can grab the leg behind the hamstring. You could also use a strap or a towel hooked around your leg. If your head doesn't rest comfortably on the floor, put something underneath it for support.

Notice whether your lower spine lifts off the floor when you pull your knee towards your chest. Try and maintain a balance between pulling the knee in and rounding the lower spine. With your lower spine flatter on the floor, you might feel more of a stretching sensation in your hip.

WHAT DOES IT DO?

Reclined pigeon particularly stretches the glutes, but also some of the deep hip muscles. This improves the capacity of the hip joint for external rotation. It can also be therapeutic for some kinds of sciatic pain and lower back problems.

WHEN YOU SHOULDN'T DO IT

If you have a knee injury that causes pain when flexing your knees, avoid this posture until the injury is resolved.

"Live each moment completely and the future will take care of itself. Fully enjoy the wonder and beauty of each moment."

PARAMAHANSA YOGANANDA

RECLINED SPINAL TWIST

Supta matsyendrasana

Because the body is fully supported by the floor, this twist works in a very different way from the seated twist. The muscles of the abdomen don't need to work so hard to hold you up, so you get an entirely different effect from the movement, and the focus for rotation is on a different part of the spine.

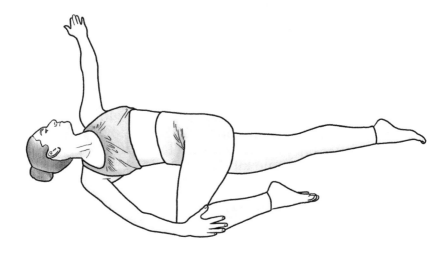

HOW TO DO IT

▷ Start lying on your back.

▷ Bend your right knee and bring it towards your chest.

▷ Draw your right knee across to the left side of your body so that your right hip lifts off the floor, allowing the spine to rotate.

▷ You can use your left hand to support the movement and bring the right knee towards the floor.

▷ Stretch your right arm out to the right on the floor at shoulder height.

▷ Turn your head to look towards the right hand.

▷ Hold the posture for 30 seconds or several long slow breaths.

▷ Repeat on the other side.

Your knee might not reach the floor - and that's fine - don't force it down. If the neck feels uncomfortable, you can keep it more neutral by not turning the head.

WHAT DOES IT DO?

Spinal twists improve the spine by keeping it mobile. They also stimulate the abdominal organs and digestive system. This version of the spinal twist stretches the glutes and balances the sacroiliac joint.

WHEN YOU SHOULDN'T DO IT

If you have a hip or a spinal injury, avoid this posture.

"Remember, it doesn't matter how deep into a posture you go. What does matter is who you are when you get there."

MAX STROM

LEGS UP THE WALL

Viparita karani

In this posture you do exactly what you'd expect from the name. You put your legs up a wall. It's a passive, supported variation of the Shoulder stand, and for this variation you'll need some sort of support like a cushion, or some folded up blankets.

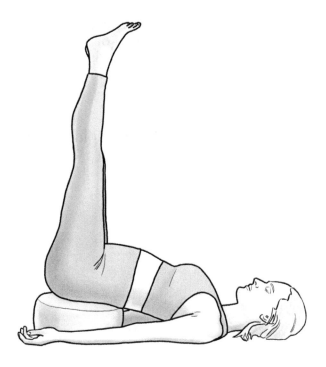

HOW TO DO IT

▷ Start lying on your back close to an open wall space.

▷ Have your support - a cushion or folded blankets - next to the wall, and your hips on the support.

▷ Lift your legs up on the wall and flex your feet so the soles face the ceiling.

▷ Readjust your position to bring your tailbone as close to the wall as possible.

- ▷ Allow the arms to fall alongside the body with the palms facing up.

- ▷ Hold the posture for a minute or longer.

This can also be practised without a support and the hips on the floor if you don't have anything suitable available.

WHAT DOES IT DO?

This kind of passive inversion helps to calm the mind - it activates the parasympathetic side of the nervous system. This has a whole load of knock-on effects and can have a really positive impact on mental health when practised consistently.

It can also help relieve tension in the lower back, and relieve tired legs and feet, especially if you have spent a lot of time in the day on your feet.

WHEN YOU SHOULDN'T DO IT:

If your hamstrings have a very limited range of motion and you can't easily lift your legs up, then you might need to start further away from the wall. If you have a bad back, be careful getting into and out of the posture.

"Yoga allows you to rediscover a sense of wholeness in your life, where you do not feel like you are constantly trying to fit broken pieces together."

BKS IYENGAR

DEAD BODY POSE

Savasana

This is usually how you'll end most practices. Some people say that it is the hardest pose to practise, even though you are doing the least. Maybe it is precisely because of that - most people try to fill their time with doing something, whether it's work, or distraction, which means doing nothing at all can be very challenging.

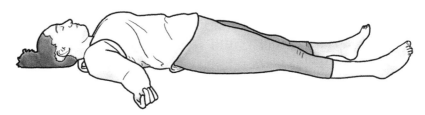

HOW TO DO IT

▷ Lie on your back with your arms by your sides and the palms facing up, the legs and the arms symmetrically spaced from the body.

▷ Close your eyes.

▷ Completely relax.

▷ Stay in the posture for as long as you want.

NOTES

If you feel uncomfortable in any part of your body, you can adjust your position and get some support. Use props to relieve any tension. For instance, if your lower back feels uncomfortable, placing a cushion or bolster underneath your knees to raise them up can help.

WHAT DOES IT DO?

This is a big question. Just like with Easy pose, *Savasana* is a jumping off point for a large part of what the practice of yoga can do for you.

The aim is to fully and completely relax your physical body while remaining in a conscious state. This has a tremendously powerful effect on the nervous system. The body and the mind are calmed, your heart rate and blood pressure go down. In the long term it can help reduce anxiety, stress, mild depression, and fatigue, while improving concentration, memory, focus, energy levels, productivity, and self-confidence. If that sounds like an unbelievable list of benefits, you only have to try it to feel its effects. Once you start to stay still and relax, everything else happens like a chain reaction.

Like all the rest, relaxation must be practised. To start with, it's not easy to lie on the floor and stay still. But if you practise it, you'll get better at doing it. Learning the art of relaxation will affect everything you experience in the rest of your life.

Savasana makes sense of everything else you do in your yoga practice. It's the counterpoint to the concentration, the balance to the effort of all the postures.

WHEN YOU SHOULDN'T DO IT

You can do Savasana any time. When you can't do anything else, you can still practise Dead body pose!

PART 3

DEVELOPING A PRACTICE

CHAPTER 12
BREATHING EXERCISES

Breathing is a fundamental part of what makes yoga work the way it does. Some of the oldest texts on yoga reference breath, and the Sanskrit term for it: *prana*. *Prana* also translates as "life force" or "energy" - which makes a lot of sense, because living things have no life when they are not breathing. Breathing exercises are often referred to as *pranayama* in yoga practice. *Yama* means "to extend," "to restrain" or "to gain control," so with these exercises you are gaining control of your energy.

According to yoga philosophy, breathing practices have a particularly beneficial effect on the subtle body, sometimes called the energy body or *pranamaya kosha*.

There's good evidence that intentional deep breathing can calm and regulate the autonomic nervous system (ANS), the system that regulates involuntary body functions such as temperature and blood pressure. Learning good breathing techniques can help ease anxiety, depression and other stress-related issues.

It is best to practise most breathing exercises or *pranayama* on an empty stomach - so if you're going to dedicate a longer practice time just for breathing, make sure it's not just after you've eaten a big meal. Exercises like square breathing can be practised anytime.

BREATHING DURING YOGA PRACTICE

The best instructions for breathing during yoga practice are quite simple.

▷ Make sure you do it.

▷ Breathe by the nose.

The first one sounds obvious, but it's just to emphasise that you shouldn't hold your breath when you're practising yoga postures. To begin with you might find both instructions difficult to follow. When you try new and often physically challenging things, it's normal to fall back on breathing patterns that you've used before in difficult situations. Holding your breath and breathing through your mouth are things which might have got you through challenging times in the past. These are habits you need to change.

So, the first step is to pay attention to how you're breathing. Try to become aware of it constantly so that you can keep it continuous and make sure you're not breathing through your mouth. Then try to make it even and regular, so that the inhale and the exhale are balanced. Try not to exhale more forcibly than you inhale or vice versa.

If you find that your breathing becomes laboured or that you start breathing through your mouth, it's a good indication to do less in the posture. Don't go as deep into your range of motion or come back to a simpler less strenuous position while you get your breath back on track.

Some people like to practise *Ujjayi* breathing (see below) when they do postures, especially if incorporating vinyasa into their practice. This can be a great way to keep the breath regulated, but it's certainly not a requirement.

OTHER KINDS OF BREATHING EXERCISE

There are many different kinds of breathing exercises that have developed throughout the course of yoga's history. The Hatha yogis used *pranayama* as a transformative practice for the energy body. If you want to explore more deeply into the tradition, it is best to find a *pranayama* teacher who has experience with the kinds of forces that extensive practice can generate in the body and mind.

All the breathing exercises below are suitable for everyone, including beginners. Always start slowly, and never force your breath. With *pranayama*, a little goes a long way. The breathing exercises should be practiced slowly and without unnecessary tension, and without ambition or any competition.

DIAPHRAGMATIC BREATHING

This is a good place to start with breathing, as it helps you to understand the mechanics of the breath. The diaphragm is the main muscle involved with breathing. It sits in the abdomen at the base of the lungs, and when you inhale it contracts and pulls down to expand the lungs.

HOW TO DO IT

▷ Start lying on your back. You can use pillows or support under your head and knees to make sure that you're comfortable.

▷ Place one hand on your upper chest.

▷ Place your other hand on your abdomen, just below the rib cage.

▷ Inhale through the nose and try to draw the breath down towards the stomach. You should feel your stomach push against the hand there, but the hand on the chest should remain relatively still.

> Exhale through the pursed lips, and slightly contract the abdominals, so that the stomach goes down. The hand on the chest should continue to remain still.

HOW LONG FOR

You can practise this for 5-10 minutes at a time.

THREE-PART BREATH

This is sometimes called the full yogic breath, and it's a good continuation from diaphragmatic breathing. The "three parts" are the diaphragm, the rib cage and the upper chest, and the aim is to consciously use as much of the lungs as possible for each breath.

HOW TO DO IT

> You can practise this breathing exercise in any comfortable position where the spine stays straight, and the abdomen is not compressed. Choose either lying down, or seated in Easy pose or Diamond pose, depending on how your knees feel, and use as much support as necessary.

> Just as with diaphragmatic breathing, place one hand on your upper chest, and place your other hand on your abdomen, just below the rib cage.

> Inhale through the nose and try to draw the breath down towards the stomach. You should feel your stomach push against the hand there.

> When you feel that the diaphragm has contracted as much as it will without forcing it, allow the ribcage to start to expand too.

> Bring the breath all the way into the upper chest so that you also feel a little bit of pressure against the hand there as the upper chest expands.

> As you exhale, reverse the process, first the air leaves the chest, then the rib cage draws back and in, and finally the belly drops completely.

> This can take a little bit of practise, but eventually you should be able to make it a smooth and continuous inhale and exhale.

HOW LONG FOR

When you're first starting out, don't overdo it, begin with 5-10 rounds. As it becomes more natural, you can increase the time to 5-10 minutes.

UJJAYI BREATH

You might have heard this called "Victorious breath" (because that's what *ujjayi* translates as), or even "Ocean breath." The sound it makes is often compared to the soft sound of the waves coming into the shore, especially when a roomful of people start practising it all together.

You can practise this kind of breathing at any time, although it is currently very popular to use Ujjayi breath when practising vinyasa yoga. It helps to create heat in the body, so it won't be suitable for all kinds of practice, especially slow, calming and restorative ones.

If it is a breathing technique that you choose to use when you practice yoga postures, you might find that it has a knock-on effect to the times outside of your practice. It can have a calming and centring effect by association of the times that you have most often used it.

HOW TO DO IT

> Start sitting in a comfortable position with the spine straight, and with as much support for your hips and knees as necessary.

> If you've never practised this breathing exercise before, the easiest way is to try it with your mouth open.

> Bring one palm in front of your mouth, with the palm facing towards your face.

▷ With your mouth open, exhale into your palm, so that you can feel your warm breath on your hand. Imagine that you are trying to fog up a mirror so your breath makes a sound in the back of your throat.

▷ Try to make the same sound in your throat on the inhale as well and practise a few breaths with the mouth open to get a feel for the sensation in the throat.

▷ You can experiment keeping your mouth open for the inhale and closed for the exhale, and vice versa, while trying to keep the same sound of your breath in the throat.

▷ Once you feel that you can move on. Bring the hand down away from your face and practise with your mouth closed.

▷ Try to keep the inhale the same length and speed as the exhale. This can take some practise as you might find either the inhale or exhale easier than the other. If one is longer than the other, make the longer one shorter to start, and then try to increase the length of both.

HOW LONG FOR

If you're using it as part of your asana practice, then use Ujjayi breathing for as long as you are practising the postures. In Savasana, you let the breath drop completely. Otherwise, you can practise the breathing exercise on its own for 5-10 minutes.

ALTERNATE NOSTRIL BREATHING

Alternate nostril breathing is often called Nadi Shodhana in Sanskrit, which literally translates as "channel purification." Nadi means "channel" and here the specific channels referred to are the ones that carry prana or energy around the subtle body.

There are several different ways of practising this kind

of breathing exercise, and different schools start with different nostrils, or on an inhale rather than an exhale. Traditionally, the breath is also practised with breath retention and fixed ratio breathing, but this is just going to be an explanation of one of the simplest ways of practising it.

You have to pay attention to which part of the cycle you are on, and to begin with can take some getting used to.

HOW TO DO IT

▷ Start sitting in a comfortable position with the spine straight, and with as much support for your hips and knees as necessary.

▷ With your right hand, bring your index finger and middle finger to rest between your eyebrows. The fingers you'll be actively using are the thumb and ring finger.

▷ Close your eyes and inhale and exhale a few breaths through your nose.

▷ After an exhale, use your right thumb to close your right nostril and slowly and steadily inhale through your left nostril.

▷ Close your left nostril with your ring finger. Open your right nostril and release the breath slowly through the right side.

▷ Inhale again through the right side. Close your right nostril with your thumb and exhale slowly through the left side.

▷ Then inhale through the left side and continue the process.

HOW LONG FOR

Start with 3-5 cycles when you are first starting out, and then breathe normally afterwards. You can increase this to 5-10 cycles with practice.

SQUARE BREATHING

Square breathing is sometimes called box breathing, and it's a great way to get started with some very simple breath retention. Gently holding your breath influences CO_2 levels in the body, which in turn affects your nervous system, slowing your heart rate. It can help reduce stress and improve your mood. This is a great breathing exercise if you suffer from anxiety.

HOW TO DO IT

▷ Start sitting in a comfortable position with the spine straight, and with as much support for your hips and knees as necessary.

▷ Inhale through the nose for a slow count of four.

▷ With the lungs completely full, hold your breath for a count of four.

▷ Exhale through the nose for a count of four.

▷ With the lungs empty, hold your breath for a count of four.

HOW LONG FOR

Start by doing 4 rounds and build up to 5-10 minutes if you want to do a longer practice. You can practise 4 rounds of it whenever you need it. If you find that a count of four doesn't feel right for you, then change the length of the breaths and retention to something more suitable.

BEE BREATHING

Bee breathing is called Brahmari Pranayama, and it gets its name from the sound you make when you exhale. It resembles the humming sound of a bee, and it can be a very relaxing and soothing breathing exercise to practise. It's ideal to do before a meditation, or last thing at night, but it can be practised at any time of day.

HOW TO DO IT

▷ Start sitting in a comfortable position with the spine straight, and with as much support for your hips and knees as necessary.

▷ Close your eyes, and keep your mouth closed, but don't clench your teeth shut.

▷ Bring your thumbs to your ears and close them - don't put your thumbs in your ears, instead close the opening by pushing the tragus cartilage (the small, pointed bit of the external ear in front of the earhole) to cover it.

▷ Spread the rest of your fingers over the crown of the head and rest them there.

▷ Breathe in slowly through your nose, and when you exhale make a low-pitched 'hmmm' at the back of your throat.

▷ Practice making the sound as smooth, and steady as you can. It doesn't need to be loud as you will be able to feel a vibration resonate through your head.

HOW LONG FOR

Practise 3-5 rounds to start with. Once you're confident with the breathing exercise, it can be practised for as long as it feels comfortable. Aim to lengthen the exhale slowly over time - but don't force it as this will create the opposite of the relaxing effect that pranayama can instil.

LION'S BREATH

This breathing exercise acts as a kind of punctuation - a way of mentally and physically separating one moment from the next. It can make you feel a bit silly or self-conscious when you do it in front of other people, but luckily, as you're reading about this in a book, you can practice it in the privacy of your own room!

HOW TO DO IT

▷ You can practise this sitting down, lying on your back, or even in any of the postures where you don't feel that your breath is too taxed by the effort, and your diaphragm can move freely.

▷ Inhale through the nose to fill the lungs.

▷ Open your mouth wide to exhale. Simultaneously stretch your tongue out, reaching the tip down toward the chin, open your eyes wide, and exhale the breath slowly out through your mouth with a distinct "ha" sound.

▷ Slightly contract the muscles on the front of your throat as you exhale and feel that the breath is passing over the back of your throat.

▷ You can use a gaze point, or drishti, for the breathing exercise. Some traditions say to look at the third eye point, some at the tip of the nose. You can even do it with your eyes closed at the end of a practice.

HOW LONG FOR

Repeat up to 6 or 7 times.

CHAPTER 13
MEDITATION

Meditation is a subject that can be covered in a single sentence, and one that can require a whole book of its own.

In Patanjali's Yoga Sutra, the 8-limbed path of yoga (see Chapter 15 - 'A (very brief) histroy of Yoga'), meditation is separate from *asana* - from posture practice - but the reality is, when you practise yoga postures, you are also practising a kind of integrated meditation. Yoga *is* meditation!

However, here we're going to briefly discuss seated meditation, because it is a practice that you can easily incorporate into a daily routine and one that you can do anywhere without any equipment. You don't even need a yoga mat. It's also a practice that will give you unexpected benefits.

WHAT CAN MEDITATION DO?

Meditation isn't a miracle cure-all, but like posture practice, can provide moments of space in your life which makes room for all sorts of marvellous and unexpected things to happen.

As well as reducing stress, controlling anxiety and promoting emotional health, meditation can do a lot more for your brain. Research has shown that meditation can lengthen your attention span, and that it can influence the tendency for the mind to wander, which unchecked often leads to worrying and poor attention.

There is also some research suggesting that meditation may have a positive effect on age-related cognitive decline and can help reduce memory loss. It can also affect addictive behaviours, helping to reduce them, including emotional and binge eating.

While meditation predominantly works on the mind, it also has the potential for creating physical changes. It can reduce blood pressure, help control pain and improve sleep.

Of course, to make the distinction between body and mind on this level almost doesn't make sense - and this is part of the big subject that yoga and meditation is all about.

HOW TO DO IT

There are actually many different styles of meditation that are popular, and in this book we are only going to look at two of them. The first is probably the most popular worldwide, which is mindfulness meditation. The second is body scan meditation, which can easily be incorporated into the end of a practice.

You can practise meditation as and when you feel like it, but a good way of making it part of your life is to establish a routine which includes it. Even just a few minutes a day can make a really big difference.

MINDFULNESS MEDITATION

Mindfulness comes from a Buddhist tradition of meditation. It's so popular because it's easy to practise on your own without a teacher. Practising it can help to bring you to a state of present moment awareness and make it easier to unravel the habitual thought patterns that can dominate your consciousness.

▷ Find a comfortable place to sit. You can do mindfulness meditation lying down, but there's a higher chance that you'll fall asleep if you're tired. Sleeping might be just what you need to do though.

▷ You can sit on a chair or sit in Easy pose. Make sure that you have enough support for your back and your knees. If you're going to sit for a long time, sit on a cushion to raise your hips a little.

▷ Choose a place that is free from distractions, where you are unlikely to be disturbed for the duration of the meditation.

▷ Set a timer - when you're first starting out, choose a short time like 5-10 minutes.

▷ Close your eyes and sit still.

▷ Follow the sensation of your breath as it goes in and out of your nose.

▷ Notice when your mind wanders and you start thinking about other things.

▷ When this happens, don't give yourself a hard time - this is the normal condition of the mind. Notice what it is you were thinking about or what was distracting you.

▷ Take a moment and pause. Let go of whatever you were thinking about.

▷ Bring your awareness back to the sensation of your breath.

▷ Continue until your timer goes off.

The practise of this kind of meditation can help you realise when your mind is overwhelmed with thoughts that you don't need to engage with. Bringing your attention back to your breath or to your awareness of the present moment is really the main skill that is being developed through the practice. Don't think that you're trying to create a mind devoid of thoughts. Your mind will be bound to wander, you just have to make the continual and compassionate effort to bring it back to a point of attention.

BODY SCAN MEDITATION

As the name suggests, body scan meditation focuses on your body. It's actually a kind of mindfulness meditation, but with more direction. It's a bit like taking a mental X-ray of your body, using your awareness as the X-ray machine. This is a great meditation to do in Dead body pose at the end of a practice if you have more time available for relaxation.

▷ You can do this sitting down, but lying down works best, so that you can stretch your arms and legs out. Make sure you're comfortable and have as much support for your body as you need.

▷ Close your eyes and open your awareness to the sensation of your breathing.

▷ Choose a point to start on in your body - it could be the left foot, right hand, top of your head, or anywhere.

▷ Focus your attention on the body part and start to become aware of any sensation you might feel. Keep breathing slowly and steadily.

▷ Acknowledge any sensation that you feel, whether it's pressure, heat, tension, discomfort or something else. Try not to associate it with anything else, just experience the sensation as it is.

▷ Stay for up to a minute or so observing the

sensations. Allow your breath to dissipate anything that needs to be released.

▷ Move onto the next area - you can do this on a breath - and start to open your awareness to the sensations there. It usually makes most sense to move onto an area that is geographically adjacent to the last (left foot to left ankle to left calf and so on) - but use a system that works for you.

▷ As with mindfulness meditation, notice when your mind wanders and you start thinking about other things. This will happen, so take a moment and pause, and let go of whatever you were thinking about.

▷ Once you have finished scanning all the parts of the body individually, take a moment to bring your awareness to the whole body simultaneously.

This meditation can have a profound effect on releasing tension in the whole body. However, try not to approach it - or any kind of meditation - with a specific goal. Instead, set out some regular time for it in your day, and take it practice by practice.

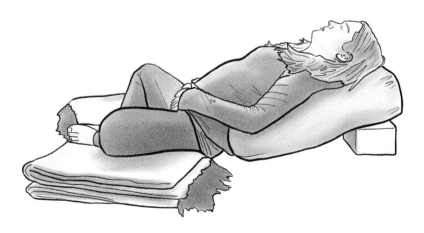

CHAPTER 14
PLANNING A PRACTICE

The simplest way to practise, at least to start with, is to follow one of the sample sequences you'll find in the back of the book. But before you do that, you can go over some of the postures in the book and become familiar with them. Go slowly and see what looks interesting or what you find easy or hard. When you want to try a sequence, if you're brand new to yoga, start with the Beginners' sequence.

WHAT KIND OF PRACTICE?

Once you've practised a few of the sequence and have some understanding of the different postures, and the sequence of a sun salutation, start to pay attention to how practising the different types of posture makes you feel.

Like learning a language, once you understand some grammar and have a bit of vocabulary, you can start putting things together yourself to come up with entirely new combinations. That way you can start practising what you need. So not only focusing on muscle groups and body parts, you can also put together a practice that helps your state of mind, your energy levels and your motivation.

For instance, if you're feeling lethargic, but you know that backbends will wake you up, you can incorporate them into a sequence if you've got things to do that you need to be more alert for. Or if you've got lots of spare time, you can repeat sections of sequences and try a different kind of focus or transition to develop your understanding of the postures.

Postures can all be practised statically, or as part of a flowing sequence, which is often referred to as vinyasa. Have a look at the section below to get a better understanding of vinyasa.

SEQUENCING

There are many different approaches you can take to sequencing a yoga asana practice, and they all have merits - there's no one right way. Part of the fun of practice can be finding unexpected connections between different movements and positions.

A standard format that is often followed is first to practise standing postures, then seated postures, then postures lying on your stomach and then ones lying on your back. This creates an arc of energy that means you are more relaxed by the end of the practice.

The way the postures have been ordered in this book is another way of sequencing that is very effective and fairly popular in Modern yoga practice. Start with warmups on the floor, like Cat-cow and Thread the needle, move on to Sun salutations, then to standing postures, like Triangle, Standing wide leg forward fold and one leg balancing poses. Once you're thoroughly warmed up, do some backbend postures, like Locust and Camel, followed by seated forward bends like Head to knee pose and finally finish with poses lying on your back, like Legs up the wall and Supine twist.

You can of course choose your own way to practise, mixing up standing and seated postures, backbends and forward bends. After all, the Sun salutations have a great variety of postures all in one package!

Ultimately, it's best to move your body in as many different ways as possible, so creating a sequence that moves all the joints and aims to strengthen all the muscles will give you the greatest benefit.

WHEN AND WHAT TO EAT BEFORE PRACTICING

This is always a big question with yoga, and it depends a lot on the individual. Traditional pranayama practice always recommends that you don't do breathing exercises after eating and should wait until there isn't food in your stomach. One of the exceptions of this is square breathing, which can be done at any time.

A lot of people can feel faint or shaky if they don't eat before practising yoga first thing in the morning, and it'll be down to you to work out what works best. Eating a lot can mean your stomach is too full, and some postures will put extra pressure on the digestive system at the wrong time. Experiment with what you eat and when you eat it to work out how to get the most out of your practice.

PRACTICE SPACE

If you can, try and dedicate an area in your home to yoga. That doesn't mean you need a whole room with all the props, posters, and incense but you can if you want! The simplest way is to lay out your yoga mat somewhere and try to keep it there. This can be hard if you don't have a lot of space, but it will mean that you are more likely to step onto it more often, even if it's only for a couple of minutes at a time. Sometimes the best and most effective practices are short and sweet.

If you dedicate an area that is specifically for yoga and you live with others, they can see that you're in that space and may be less likely to disturb you. That isn't always possible with young children! However, associating space with action and intentions can have a powerful effect, even on little ones.

FOCUS

Try to practise distraction free. This can be difficult – again, especially if you have young children. Apart from unavoidable distractions, try to create a space of focus to practise in. That means whenever possible, turn off your phone and try not to look at it, let people you live with know that they shouldn't disturb you, and play music rather than listen to a podcast. Don't have the TV on in the background! You can also practise in silence, just to the sound of your breath...

In most of the postures there's some instruction of where to look when you're holding the pose. This is the essence of an idea called *drishti*, which can be translated as "focused gaze." Try to keep your eyes on a fixed point during the posture. It doesn't have to be the one described in the instructions, especially if using it makes your neck feel uncomfortable. Notice if your eyes move around a lot and try to bring them back again and again to the point of focused gaze.

VINYASA

Vinyasa yoga is probably the most popular form of yoga in the world at the moment. It's a style that has many different formats and traditions associated with it: Ashtanga Vinyasa, Rocket Yoga, Power Yoga, Jivamukti Yoga all use the vinyasa form, as well as countless other yoga classes in yoga studios everywhere.

The basis of the style is that you transition between postures of a sequence by combining the movement with your breath. For this reason, some people refer to it as "breath-movement yoga."

For instance, a very simple example: stand in Mountain pose and, as you inhale, sweep your arms up over your head into Upwards arms pose and, as you exhale, bring your arms back down into Mountain pose. This would be vinyasa.

You can practise this with lots of different movements: you can bend and straighten your front leg in Warrior 2 - inhale as you straighten, exhale as you bend; or go from Forward fold to Half forward fold on an inhale and back down again on an exhale.

Breath-movement lends itself ideally to Sun salutations, and they are most well-known for using vinyasa. This gives the practice a certain sense of timing - all the movements take the same amount of time - as you try to regulate the breath to be even throughout. As the distance the body travels is greater between some postures than others, sometimes you'll need to move faster than others, even though the speed of the breath stays the same.

Quite often the combination of Low-level plank, Upward dog and Downward dog will be called "a vinyasa." Traditionally, in the style called Ashtanga Vinyasa, this combination of postures is practised in between every single posture which not only helps to develop strength but keeps the pace of the practice regular and meditative.

You can also practise other postures in a sequence using vinyasa transitions. For instance, from Warrior 2, you could inhale and straighten your front leg, and exhale, stretch your front arm forward and bring it down onto your front leg into Triangle pose. From Triangle pose, you could inhale and bring your torso back to an upright position and then exhale, bend your front knee again, and bring your hand to the floor beside the front foot for Side angle.

There's a sample sequence below of a simple vinyasa with some instructions for the transitions. However, one of the best ways of getting a feel for how to make the transitions work is to practise the individual postures in the book, and experiment with some movements which you link to your breathing. See what feels natural, and what doesn't. See whether the movement might take you into another posture, or whether it's just one that is self-contained within the posture itself.

CHAPTER 15

A (VERY BRIEF) HISTORY OF YOGA

Yoga's had a lot of different definitions throughout its life. Most commonly now you will hear the definition, "Yoga is union," often derived from the Sanskrit root of the word *yuj* which means "to attach, join, harness, yoke." The union can be between any two apparently separate things: the mind and the body, the body and the soul, the individual consciousness and the cosmic consciousness, you and the universe.

When it first appears in the texts of yoga, specifically the *Rig Veda*, the earliest text that mentions yoga, the word means "to yoke," referring to the yoke you would place on an animal to attach it to a plough. The idea of yoga as a union is actually a relatively modern idea.

Yoga didn't appear fully formed in the way that we practise it now. There are a lot of things that many people associate with yoga, like yoga postures, or the *chakras*, or veganism, or chanting, and when you look at the history of yoga, you can start to see when and where some of the ideas have come from.

HOW OLD IS YOGA?

This is the first question to think about. Most often the figure that is passed about is 5000 years old. That might lead you to believe that the yoga presented in this book or that is practised in yoga studios around the world today looks exactly like it did 5000 years ago. The kind of yoga we practise now is usually called Modern Yoga (see below) and is quite different from what might have been practised then.

The figure of 5000 years is used because of the mention of the word "yoga" in the *Rig Veda*, which was written down in about the 15th Century BCE. That's not quite five thousand years ago, but it would have come from a much older oral tradition. All we've got to go on is the written record, so it's actually very hard to say anything with any real conviction, and even the written record is hard to date. We have to make do with approximations.

We do know that by about the 5th Century BC, yoga had started to evolve as a system of thought. When it's mentioned in the *Katha Upanishad*, it's described as follows: "When the five senses, along with the mind, remain still and the intellect is not active, that is known as the highest state." This describes a state of mind that is equivalent to a state of yoga, and so far, nothing has been mentioned about yoga postures.

YOGA OF ACTION AND YOGA OF LOVE

Thought to be written in around the 2nd Century BCE, the *Bhagavad Gita* is considered one of the holy scriptures of Hinduism. It consists of a conversation between Krishna, an avatar of the god Vishnu, and a prince called Arjuna. Krishna is Arjuna's charioteer, and they are about to charge into a battle in which the prince will have to fight and kill many members of his own family.

Krishna explains many different ideas about yoga and situates yoga as a practice that is suitable and appropriate for everyone. He associates it with non-attachment, "Be equal minded in both success and failure. Such equanimity is called Yoga." The yoga he talks about isn't an abstract meditation system, but rather real-world involvement. "Yoga is skill in action." He explains karma yoga, which is the yoga of selfless action: a true yogi is someone who works to help others and does so without any thought of a reward.

He also talks about bhakti yoga or devotional yoga. The devotion or love that he is referring to is primarily devotion to the Supreme Being (of which he is a manifestation, or *avatar*), but love is a universal experience. In love, you become selfless. Instead of giving prominence to your own desire, you consider the one you love first. This selflessness is the essence of spiritual practice.

THE YOGA OF THE YOGA SUTRA

There have been many descriptions of the methods of how to achieve this state of yoga, but one of the most popular and enduring comes from the *Yoga Sutra*. It was compiled roughly a century after the *Katha Upanishad* in the 4th Century BCE by the sage Patanjali. Like the *Katha Upanishad*, yoga is described as a state of mind: *yogas chitta vritti nirodhah*. "Yoga is the cessation of the fluctuations of the mind." Sometimes the yoga system laid out in the *Yoga Sutra* is called Classical Yoga, Eight-limbed (or Ashtanga) Yoga or even Raja Yoga (*raja* means "royal").

It's often called Eight-limbed yoga because it details eight steps - although to call them steps suggest they are sequential, and usually several of the different steps or limbs are practised concurrently. The yoga of Patanjali is best described as "concentration," or even "discipline," as the text describes a system of compounding of concentration that ultimately transforms the very mind of the practitioner.

The eight limbs are as follows:

◇ **YAMA** Moral imperatives
◇ **NIYAMA** Positive habits

- ◇ **ASANA** Posture (here probably meaning "seat", the seat of meditation)
- ◇ **PRANAYAMA** Breathing exercises (breath regulation)
- ◇ **PRATYAHARA** Sense withdrawal
- ◇ **DHARANA** Concentration
- ◇ **DHYANA** Meditation
- ◇ **SAMADHI** Oneness with the subject of meditation

The *Yamas* are ethical vows that the yogi undertakes that help contribute to their personal growth and they consist of:

AHIMSA which means "nonviolence" and extends to non-harming other living beings through actions and speech. This is why a lot of people who practise yoga for a long time become vegan.

SATYA which means truthfulness

ASTEYA which means non-stealing

BRAHMACARYA which is often translated as chastity and is now usually interpreted to mean sexual fidelity in the Western version of Modern Yoga.

APARIGRAHA which means non-possessiveness

If the *Yamas* look like a list of things you shouldn't do if you want to be a good yogi, then the *Niyamas* are the opposite. They are a list of a set of behaviours that the yogi needs to adopt.

SAUCHA which means purity, and refers to how you treat your body, mind and environment.

SANTOSHA which means contentment, a very different quality from happiness.

TAPAS translates literally to fire or heat. In this context it means something more like austerity or discipline. The fire that keeps you going on the path.

SVADHYAYA which means self-study or self-reflection, but also study of the texts of yoga.

ISHVARAPRANIDHANA which means contemplation of, or surrender to, the Supreme Being.

The *Yamas* and *Niyamas* are the context within which all the other limbs of yoga can operate, the context that will make the practice of yoga successful. The yoga of the *Yoga Sutra* is primarily a meditation system, and the eighth limb, *Samadhi*, describes the state in which there is no distinction between the meditator, the act of meditation and the subject of meditation.

HATHA YOGA

So far, all the yoga that has been covered bears very little resemblance to the yoga that's been laid out in this book. This all changes with Hatha Yoga. The main texts of Hatha Yoga are medieval, from about the 15th Century CE. As well as information about meditation, they also detail *asana* and *pranayama*. In the *Yoga Sutra*, *asana* was literally the seat of meditation, but in the Hatha Yoga texts, they are explanations for some of the yoga postures that are still popular now. Breathing exercises were expanded upon, and cleansing exercises were also explained.

The schools of Hatha yoga were an offshoot of Tantrism, esoteric traditions of Hinduism and Buddhism that developed from the middle of the 1st millennium CE. It was from Tantra that Hatha Yoga adapted and systematised many of the ideas which are still popular in yoga today. For instance, although *chakras* are an old idea and are mentioned in some of the earliest texts, Hatha yogis explained the methodology behind using them as a means of transformation.

According to the texts, *prana* permeates everything - it's a kind of lifeforce or spirit-energy. In humans it travels around the body in specialised energy channels. Chakras are energy centres in the body, created at the points where two of the main energy channels in the body cross. They are both a means of unlocking the potential energy systems in the body and mind, and a kind of meditation aid that focuses psychosomatic energy at different points in the body. In the last century, they've been added to and elaborated into a whole system that isn't exactly how they were first envisioned but has been made very compelling.

MODERN YOGA

The kind of yoga that is practised now, the kind of yoga that is detailed in this book, is often referred to as Modern Yoga. It is a synthesis of all the different yoga traditions that have come before it, with some parts removed, and more added.

Modern yoga is derived from Hatha Yoga, and in large part, yoga owes its current popularity to a teacher called Krishnamacharya. He helped fuse gymnastics into the practices of Hatha Yoga, and among his students were two widely influential teachers, Pattabhi Jois and BKS Iyengar whose yoga systems are practised all over the world. Pattabhi Jois taught Ashtanga Vinyasa Yoga, which developed into all the different vinyasa-based practices. Iyengar taught - among many things - a methodology for precise postural alignment, and the use of support and props, which has developed into restorative yoga and some of the practices of yoga therapy.

In many ways, yoga has transitioned from a purely spiritual practice to one that is focused on health and fitness. Of course, there is still a spiritual tradition running through it all, and it is important to recognise where the practice has come from, because this will ultimately give us a greater understanding of what it can do.

CHAPTER 16
SEQUENCES

There is an endless combination of different postures and their variations, and ways of transitioning between them. The following are just a few ideas. Ultimately, I hope you use this book to practise in your own unique way, to express the essence of yourself. To begin with, some guidance can be useful, so practise these sequences until you feel confident to do your own thing. You can also combine your favourite parts of the sequences together to make longer routines.

The time underneath each posture is just a recommendation for the time to hold it. If the chart recommends '30s – each side' then do that, the right side followed straight away by the left side. Alternatively, it will state '30s – R' which means you should do just the right side, and then you'll go back to do the left side later in the sequence. If you see instruction 'transition', then you don't need to hold it, you go straight onto the next posture. If there are a pair of revolving arrows, and underneath a multiplier then alternate between the two postures – for instance when you do Cat-cow.

The timings for all the sequences are all approximate – it really depends how long you stay in each posture. As you become more proficient and comfortable in the practice, feel free to stay longer in each of the postures.

BEGINNING SEQUENCE - 20 mins

This is a great sequence to get started with, working mainly on standing postures which are usually more accessible to beginners, as well as on some shoulder openers.

MORNING JUMP START - 12 mins

If you want a quick way to start your day, this is a great sequence to get all the joints moving and the blood pumping. It covers all the bases with some balancing, hip mobility and backward bending.

SIMPLE VINYASA - 30 mins

This sequence takes you through a large portion of the postures presented in this book. The intention is to practise it in vinyasa style, where you link the breath to the movements that you make. For a more in-depth description of vinyasa, have a look at the previous chapter.

ENERGY BOOST - 10 mins

For when you need a quick pick-me-up, this sequence will get your spine moving and feeling great! It's a great one to practise when you've been sitting for a long stretch, as you start by opening up and mobilising the shoulders.

STRENGTH BUILDER - 12 mins

This sequence helps you build strength -progressively adding more challenging variations of the same posture, so you can easily scale it down to start with – or make it harder if you find it gets too easy!

QUICK HAMSTRING STRETCH - 9 mins

When I tell them that I'm a yoga teacher, so many people tell me that they have tight hamstrings! Here's a great way to start getting your hamstrings more flexible. It starts with a bit of mobilisation and active stretching, so that the longer holds are more effective.

MOVE YOUR HIPS - 15 mins

In yoga the hips carry special significance because they are the base of your spine, home of the root chakra, the lowest energy centre in the body. Keeping your hips strong and flexible will go a long way to make your spine feel good – and this sequence does exactly that.

EVENING RESTORE - 15 mins

This is just simply a way of winding things down at the end of the day. Add any extra postures to this that you like that don't involve a lot of exertion and hold them for a minute or more.

BEGINNING SEQUENCE

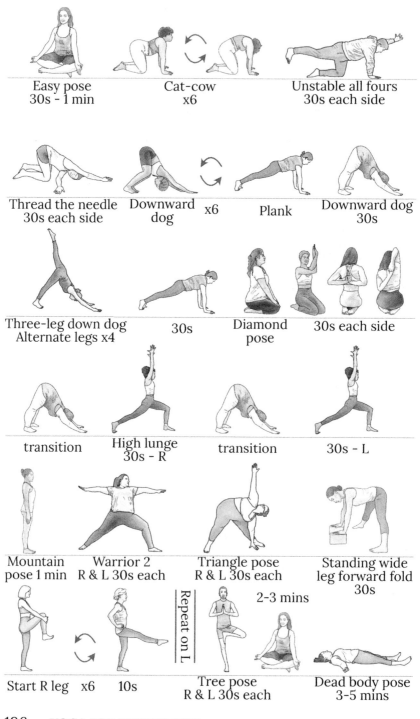

Easy pose
30s - 1 min

Cat-cow
x6

Unstable all fours
30s each side

Thread the needle
30s each side

Downward dog x6

Plank

Downward dog
30s

Three-leg down dog
Alternate legs x4

30s

Diamond pose

30s each side

transition

High lunge
30s - R

transition

30s - L

Mountain
pose 1 min

Warrior 2
R & L 30s each

Triangle pose
R & L 30s each

Standing wide
leg forward fold
30s

Start R leg   x6   10s

Repeat on L

Tree pose
R & L 30s each

2-3 mins

Dead body pose
3-5 mins

MORNING JUMP START

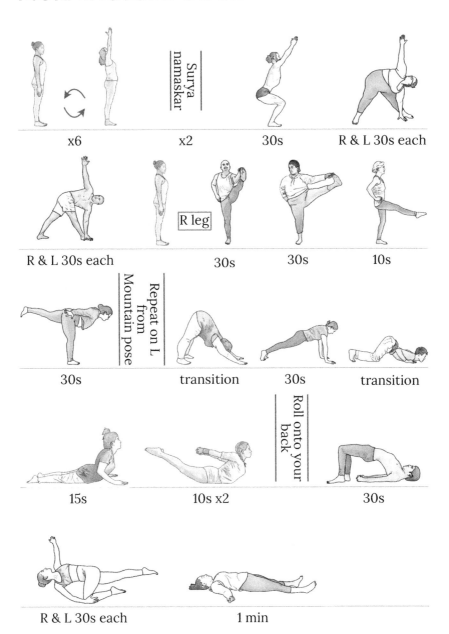

x6	x2 *Surya namaskar*	30s	R & L 30s each	
R & L 30s each	30s *R leg*	30s	10s	
30s *Repeat on L from Mountain pose*	transition	30s	transition	
15s	10s x2 *Roll onto your back*	30s		
R & L 30s each	1 min			

SIMPLE VINYASA

Instead of measuring time in minutes and seconds, in a vinyasa, you use the breath count to time how long you hold each posture.

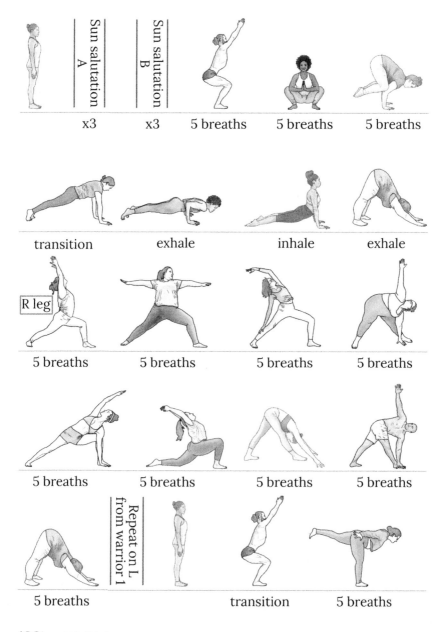

	Sun salutation A	Sun salutation B			
	x3	x3	5 breaths	5 breaths	5 breaths

transition	exhale	inhale	exhale

R leg			
5 breaths	5 breaths	5 breaths	5 breaths

5 breaths	5 breaths	5 breaths	5 breaths

5 breaths	Repeat on L from warrior 1	transition	5 breaths

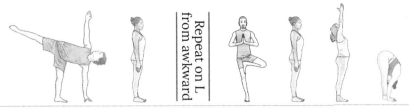

5 breaths | Repeat on L from awkward | R & L 5 breaths

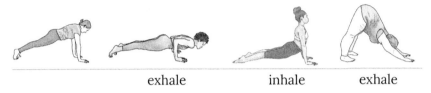

exhale inhale exhale

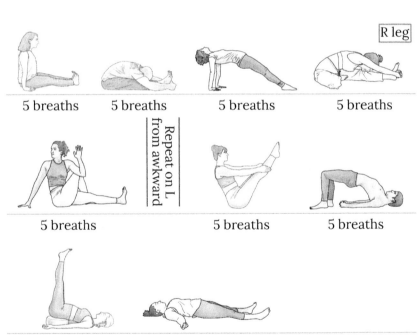

R leg

5 breaths 5 breaths 5 breaths 5 breaths

Repeat on L from awkward

5 breaths 5 breaths 5 breaths

25 breaths 3-5 mins

ENERGY BOOST

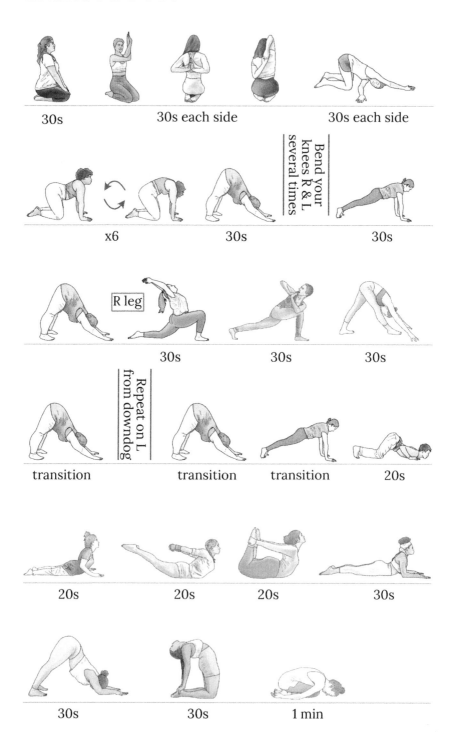

30s   30s each side   30s each side

x6   30s   Bend your knees R & L several times   30s

R leg

30s   30s   30s

transition   Repeat on L from downdog   transition   transition   20s

20s   20s   20s   30s

30s   30s   1 min

STRENGTH BUILDER

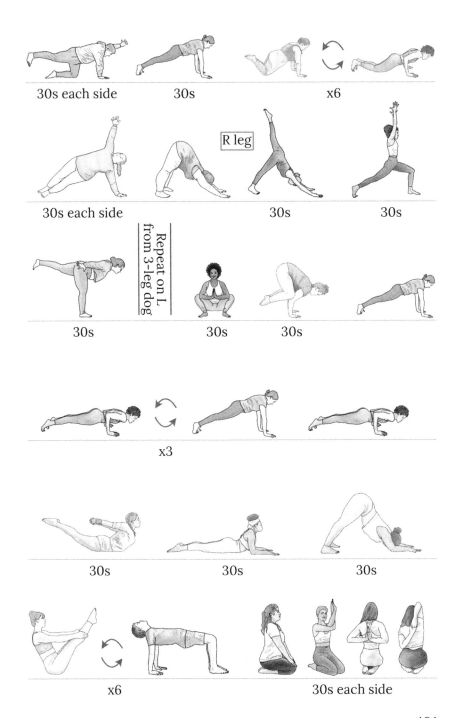

30s each side   30s   x6

R leg

30s each side   30s   30s

Repeat on L from 3-leg dog

30s   30s   30s

x3

30s   30s   30s

x6   30s each side

191

QUICK HAMSTRING STRETCH

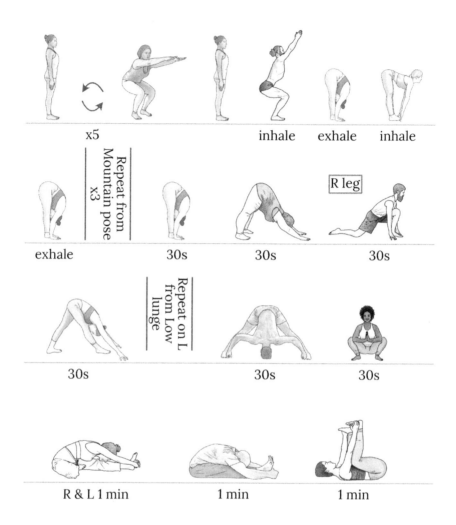

x5

inhale   exhale   inhale

Repeat from Mountain pose x3

exhale   30s   30s   30s

R leg

Repeat on L from Low lunge

30s   30s   30s

R & L 1 min   1 min   1 min

MOVE YOUR HIPS

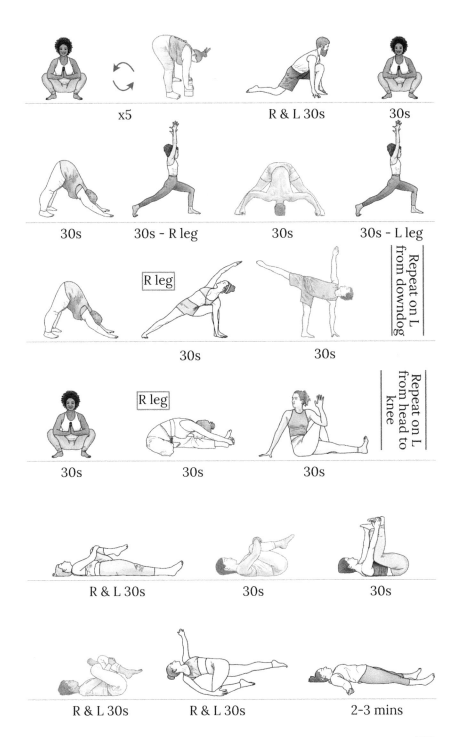

x5   R & L 30s   30s

30s   30s - R leg   30s   30s - L leg

R leg   Repeat on L from downdog

30s   30s

R leg   Repeat on L from head to knee

30s   30s   30s

R & L 30s   30s   30s

R & L 30s   R & L 30s   2-3 mins

193

EVENING RESTORE

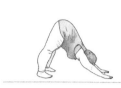

R & L 1 min   1 min

  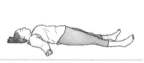

1 min   R & L 1 min   1 min

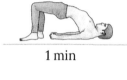 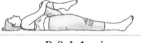

1 min   3 mins   3-5 mins

A NOTE FROM THE AUTHOR

I really hope you've enjoyed the information contained within this book. It is the culmination of my many years of teaching and practising yoga. It not only contains the postures and exercises that I think it's best to get started with in your practice, but also the ones that can provide the foundation for your practice for the rest of your life.

Yoga doesn't need to be extravagant or complicated to be effective. You don't need to do "advanced" postures to reap the benefits. All you have to do is show up. Be consistent. Take it one day at a time, one step at time and one breath at a time.

I'd really appreciate hearing what you think about the book as I always want to improve what I'm offering, so if you'd consider leaving me a review that would be tremendously appreciated.

With all love,

LUISA RAY

REFERENCES

The following is a selection of references for the information contained within this book. Of course, a lot more went into the writing of it, from the countless books I've read over the course of my yoga career, to the trainings I've attended and the teachings I've received. This is by no means an extensive bibliography. However, the journals which provided some of the scientific basis of what I've included are listed below, as well some of the key texts.

BENEFITS OF YOGA

Katuri, K. K., Dasari, A. B., Kurapati, S., Vinnakota, N. R., Bollepalli, A. C., & Dhulipalla, R. (2016). Association of yoga practice and serum cortisol levels in chronic periodontitis patients with stress-related anxiety and depression. *Journal of International Society of Preventive & Community Dentistry*, 6(1), 7–14. https://doi.org/10.4103/2231-0762.175404

García-Sesnich, J. N., Flores, M. G., Ríos, M. H., & Aravena, J. G. (2017). Longitudinal and Immediate Effect of Kundalini Yoga on Salivary Levels of Cortisol and Activity of Alpha-Amylase and Its Effect on Perceived Stress. *International journal of yoga*, 10(2), 73–80. https://doi.org/10.4103/ijoy.IJOY_45_16

Hofmann, S. G., Andreoli, G., Carpenter, J. K., & Curtiss, J. (2016). Effect of Hatha Yoga on Anxiety: A Meta-

Analysis. Journal of evidence-based medicine, 9(3), 116–124. https://doi.org/10.1111/jebm.12204

Djalilova, D. M., Schulz, P. S., Berger, A. M., Case, A. J., Kupzyk, K. A., & Ross, A. C. (2019). Impact of Yoga on Inflammatory Biomarkers: A Systematic Review. Biological Research For Nursing, 21(2), 198–209. https://doi.org/10.1177/1099800418820162

Wieland LS, Skoetz N, Pilkington K, Vempati R, D'Adamo CR, Berman BM. Yoga treatment for chronic non-specific low back pain. Cochrane Database of Systematic Reviews 2017, Issue 1. Art. No.: CD010671. DOI: 10.1002/14651858.CD010671.pub2. Accessed 30 July 2021.

Russell, Natalie DPT; Daniels, Bevin PT, DPT; Smoot, Betty PT, DPTSc; Allen, Diane D. PT, PhD Effects of Yoga on Quality of Life and Pain in Women With Chronic Pelvic Pain: Systematic Review and Meta-Analysis, Journal of Women's Health Physical Therapy: July/September 2019 - Volume 43 - Issue 3 - p 144-154 doi: 10.1097/JWH.0000000000000135

Datta, K., Tripathi, M. & Mallick, H.N. *Yoga Nidra*: An innovative approach for management of chronic insomnia- A case report. *Sleep Science Practice* **1,** 7 (2017). https://doi.org/10.1186/s41606-017-0009-4

Polsgrove, M. J., Eggleston, B. M., & Lockyer, R. J. (2016). Impact of 10-weeks of yoga practice on flexibility and balance of college athletes. *International Journal of Yoga*, 9(1), 27–34. https://doi.org/10.4103/0973-6131.171710

Halder, K., Chatterjee, A., Pal, R., Tomer, O. S., & Saha, M. (2015). Age related differences of selected Hatha yoga practices on anthropometric characteristics, muscular strength and flexibility of healthy individuals. *International journal of yoga*, 8(1), 37–46. https://doi.org/10.4103/0973-6131.146057

Apar Avinash Saoji, B.R. Raghavendra, N.K. Manjunath, (2019) Effects of yogic breath regulation: A narrative review of scientific evidence, Journal of Ayurveda and

Integrative Medicine, Volume 10, Issue 1, Pages 50-58, https://doi.org/10.1016/j.jaim.2017.07.008.

Hunter S, Laosiripisan J, Elmenshawy A, Tanaka H. Effects of yoga interventions practised in heated and thermoneutral conditions on endothelium-dependent vasodilatation: The Bikram yoga heart study. *Experimental Physiology* 2018, https://doi.org/10.1113/EP086725

Sharma P, Poojary G, Dwivedi SN, Deepak KK. Effect of Yoga-Based Intervention in Patients with Inflammatory Bowel Disease. *Int J Yoga Therap.* 2015;25(1):101-12. doi: 10.17761/1531-2054-25.1.101. Erratum in: Int J Yoga Therap. 2016 Jan;26(1):131. PMID: 26667293.

A. Ross, A. Brooks, K. Touchton-Leonard, G. Wallen, (2016), "A Different Weight Loss Experience: A Qualitative Study Exploring the Behavioral, Physical, and Psychosocial Changes Associated with Yoga That Promote Weight Loss", *Evidence-Based Complementary and Alternative Medicine*, vol. 2016, . https://doi.org/10.1155/2016/2914745

POSTURES

Iyengar, B. K. S, (1979), *Light on Yoga: The Bible of Modern Yoga*
Maehle, G, (2007), *Ashtanga Yoga: Practice and Philosophy*

MEDITATION

Norris, C. J., Creem, D., Hendler, R., & Kober, H. (2018). Brief Mindfulness Meditation Improves Attention in Novices: Evidence From ERPs and Moderation by Neuroticism. *Frontiers in human neuroscience*, 12, 315. https://doi.org/10.3389/fnhum.2018.00315

Sood A, Jones DT. On mind wandering, attention, brain networks, and meditation. *Explore* (NY). 2013 May-Jun;9(3):136-41. doi: 10.1016/j.explore.2013.02.005. PMID: 23643368.

Gard T, Hölzel BK, Lazar SW. The potential effects of meditation on age-related cognitive decline: a systematic review. *Ann N Y Acad Sci.* 2014 Jan;1307:89-103. doi: 10.1111/nyas.12348. PMID: 24571182; PMCID: PMC4024457.

Katterman SN, Kleinman BM, Hood MM, Nackers LM, Corsica JA. Mindfulness meditation as an intervention for binge eating, emotional eating, and weight loss: a systematic review. *Eat Behav.* 2014 Apr;15(2):197-204. doi: 10.1016/j.eatbeh.2014.01.005. Epub 2014 Feb 1. PMID: 24854804.

Koike MK, Cardoso R. Meditation can produce beneficial effects to prevent cardiovascular disease. *Horm Mol Biol Clin Investig.* 2014 Jun;18(3):137-43. doi: 10.1515/hmbci-2013-0056. PMID: 25390009.

HISTORY OF YOGA

Easwaran, E (2007), *The Bhagavad Gita, 2nd Edition*
Sri Swami Satchidananda, (2012), *The Yoga Sutras of Patanjali*
Simpson, D, (2021), *The Truth of Yoga: A Comprehensive Guide to Yoga's History, Texts, Philosophy, and Practices*

POSTURE INDEX

ACKNOWLEDGEMENTS

This kind of thing normally goes at the front of the book – where you thank everyone who has helped in its creation, but I wanted it to be easy to find so that I can continue to express my gratitude to those who have been so instrumental in making this all possible.

First and foremost, I need to thank the teacher who saw the teacher in me, Yogacharya Anand Prakash, who taught me on my first teacher training. He was an amazing man who helped to infuse my practice with joy and inspired me to share the teachings of yoga with as many people as I could. And I must thank my friend, Monica, who took me to my first class so many years ago. Without her I don't know where I would be now.

Angus has done amazing work with all the illustrations. I want to thank my friends and students for their patience in posing for the postures, and for their input into what they thought was important for a beginner at yoga to know and understand. Thanks to my editors, Mary and Emilio, and to everyone at Vital Life Books for their patience and belief in me.

Printed in Great Britain
by Amazon

21398649R00120